Mindful Dementia Care

Mindful Dementia Care

*Lost and Found in
the Alzheimer's Forest*

Ruth Dennis
with Velma Arellano and
Luke Nachtrab

Golden Word Books
Santa Fe, NM

Published by Golden Word Books, Santa Fe, New Mexico.

ISBN 978-1-948749-14-5

Dedicated to the countless number of elders, families, friends, and neighbors near and far who have entrusted us to walk through this forest with them over the past twenty years. We have shared great food, laughs, tears, and stories.

May I be protector to those without protection?
A leader for those who journey,
And a boat, a passage
For those desiring the further shore

May the pain of every living creature
Be completely cleared away.
May I be the doctor and the medicine.
And may I be nurse
For all sick beings in the world
Until everyone is healed.

Just like space
And the greatest elements such as earth,
May I always support the life of all boundless creatures.

And until they pass away from pain
May I also be a source of life
For all the realms of varied beings
That reach unto the ends of space.

—Sogyal Rinpoche, *The Tibetan Book of Living and Dying*

Contents

Introduction

The idea of writing this book has been a shared dream for more than ten years now. So far, life and being a caregiver both professionally and personally have caused "the book" to be an ever-present future plan. Oddly enough, it is an increase in the deeply personal side of caregiving for me that has allowed me to start "the book." The best place to start seems to be saying what this project is *not* and what it could become.

While twenty years of my professional life have been devoted to being, in many forms, a caregiver to elders facing dementia, this is not a clinical study of memory loss or a resource guide to dementia—or Down syndrome (I will explain this shortly). Nor is it a palliative care or hospice care manual. Instead, my hope is that by sharing information and stories, this book will encourage all of us to celebrate hope for the people we love and examine questions and dreams for making the future better for elders, families, and caregivers of all kinds. I hope it can offer ways to take a careful, practical, and loving look at how all of us as caregivers—and care receivers—make decisions about care. What part of us is really driving the bus when we make decisions in the most difficult times of life? It is also a call to pay attention, to value the time we have, and to learn from those around us who have a different vision of the world we all share.

The intersection of my professional and personal life is the Vista Living Care community. For the past nineteen years, Vista has been an adventure, a place to learn and grow where

I have had the privilege of being the social services director. My role is to provide support and education for families facing all forms of dementia.

Sierra Vista Alzheimer's Community was the first assisted living in the great state of New Mexico to be inducted into the Eden Alternative Registry. Eden Alternative is the honor society for long-term care dedicated to transforming the culture of care; being a part of this registry makes a public statement about our commitment to the journey of change. In 2016, I was blessed to present at the International Eden Alternative Conference on the arts and healing in dementia care. Eden Alternative and the ideas that come out of this movement will come up throughout this book.

The support that our Vista family has received from this movement has been a great learning experience. We value our elders through creating a home that honors the whole person. Our elders' lives are rich, and our home is filled with art, animal companions, music, dance, books, laughter, and wholesome food. We embrace the goal of creating a more loving, spiritual approach to aging for all elders and their families. Using the creative artistic process to achieve these goals has been the focus of my working life for the past twenty years. The elders, caregivers, families, and friends—for myself and my brother Morgan—are *family*.

Velma Arellano has been Morgan's "other sister" for these seventeen years and is both a co-creator of this book and the rock of the Vista Living Care family. She and my friend Linda Allen are a deeply honest and devoted—and at times annoying!—family for Morgan and me.

Morgan, who is 51 at the time of this writing, lives with me, has Down syndrome, and has always been the greatest teacher in my life. He is an artist and a musician and has a deep loving connection to animals, children, and elders. Morgan (also called "the Dude") has an encyclopedic knowledge for all things science fiction and a love of all kinds of music, from

Segovia to Guns and Roses. He is also the single bravest human being I have ever known.

Jude Thomas, who cofounded the Eden Alternative, uses a phrase I dearly love to describe the idea that a person can be a place of rest and grounding for another: "human sanctuary." In the work we do at Vista Living Care, our hope is to always be this for elders and families. Yet I did not give much thought to where my own "human sanctuary" was, until now. Morgan is that for me. He shares love, he is stubborn, creative, and fearless, and he is dying. All the years of working with elders and families wash away when someone I love needs a very different kind of care. There is a profound difference between the knowledge of caregiving and the soul who lives with this each day.

The truth is I am one of many facing this. Almost all of the beautiful people I work with are also family caregivers in some form. The youngest are caregivers for children or teen-agers. The rest care for aging parents, grandchildren, disabled siblings, spouses who face chronic illness, and often more than one of these at the same time.

The National Alliance for Caregiving and AARP released a joint study in 2015 that found 43.5 million people in the United States were caregivers; of those, 33 million were caring for other adults, and 6.8 million were caring for both children and adults. According to the Alzheimer's Association, 5.7 million people face Alzheimer's disease, and 16.1 million people provide unpaid care for them, which is valued at more than $232 billion per year. The Centers for Disease Control estimates that 70 percent of all adults in the United States over the age of 65 will need hands-on care in their lifetimes, and the World Health Organization predicts that the number of people needing daily hands-on care will triple by 2050.

Facing these numbers can be overwhelming. Knowing that there are very human stories behind each one of America's 43.5 million caregivers and each of the people they care for is a way to honor, respect, and help create systems that make these lives better. Our shared experience as human beings is to both give care and need care from one another. Living with my brother all my life has taught me that the place where positive change begins is the individual human story each one of us can share with the world. It is in the stories of individuals and families—the day-to-day heroism—that ideas to build a better future reside.

Many physicians who see themselves as patient advocates do not consider the well-being of the people doing the hands-on care. Likewise, some advocates for individuals with developmental disabilities and dementia focus so carefully on their positive, creative potential that they ignore sadness, anger, and frustration. People do act out, people do have pain, and they do feel profound loss; downplaying this is not respectful to the whole person.

A caregiver's job can be the most fulfilling in the world, but it can also be the most exhausting and the most disregarded on Earth. All the support groups and self-care advice in the world cannot create more hours in the day or more money in the bank for a family caregiver who is needing sleep and wondering how to pay the next set of bills. There is no magic way to make the decision of when to place a loved one in a facility easy. There is no simple answer to care.

Embracing the idea of a "partnership in care" is a good start, and the Eden Alternative does this. However, in this book I have made the choice to use the term "caregiver" instead of "care partner," which is the Eden term. "Caregiver" is a more accurate statement of how so many people feel and live. This word expresses the commitment one makes to give love and help to another person, often despite the personal cost involved. There is a need for all parts of care to be explored in an honest and balanced way.

My hope for this book is that in the sharing of stories and exploring of questions, we can help create a deeper and more balanced way to view care and to meet the heroic, creative, and incredibly strong people who both need and give care. (To preserve privacy, many names have been changed or omitted.) All of those millions of stories express the range of human experience. We all learn from being cared for and from caring for others. One of my dear friends who is a caregiver for her brother expressed it this way: "He taught me to LOVE."

What else is there to learn?

With Gratitude

The concept of right livelihood is one of the basic tenets of Buddhism, the idea that we should seek to provide for ourselves in ways that improve the lives of the people and world that we all share. Making the choice to work in a field that provides care, creates safety, or encourages people is to begin a path of right livelihood by contributing to a viable, sustainable environment that adds love to the world. I am blessed to have been given the opportunity to do the work I have done for the past nineteen years. I am also deeply blessed to have this time to step back from the work to reflect on the nature of caregiving and the impact it has on all of us.

The majority of my adult life has been spent working full-time and caregiving full-time, an experience that is not unique. I know how to be tired. I have faced mountains of paperwork that did little other than frustrate my brother and me. I have yelled, cried, and pushed for more options for his life and more rest in mine. I have been in awe of the amazing person my brother is. I also grieve deeply and daily for the changes he faces.

During the past year, I have increasingly gone from working the second shift of being a caregiver at home to also working the third shift of disrupted sleep as my brother's health needs changed. This forced a shift. There was a point where my body and concentration could not keep up. Many families go through this.

However, my situation is unique in a different sense. In writing and researching this book, I have realized that it is actually quite unusual—odd, even—to be part of a system that actually functions well for elders, caregivers, and families. Compassionate common sense is a rare commodity. The Vista ecosystem, while evolving, is innately healthy; sadly, this is far more unusual than it should be. Morgan and I are blessed, and I am blessed with the time and support to explore these issues through this book.

The people who have created the Vista ecosystem of care are many things in my life. They are family. Family for me is a choice, a decision. The following people are all a wonderful part of that choice, and have made this book possible.

The late Mary Arellano, a beautiful, independent, amazing woman who not only raised three of the most incredible women I have ever known, but gave her love and prayers freely to all of our extended Vista family. Your spirit and memory will always be with us.

Velma Arellano, who has been a friend, sister, co-writer, source of arguments, and a counterpoint to many of the ideas explored in this book, I am grateful for your pushing me to keep thinking—and not to overthink.

Luke Nachtrab, thank you, because you were always there. You have been willing to lead and to follow this Vista ecosystem in all its beautiful and often confusing, painful, and funny incarnations. Our particular ecosystem of care in the Vista family begins with another family. That family is yours.

Linda Allen because being there and being positive makes a difference. Your faith is appreciated. So is the fact that you really love grammar and sentence structure.

Morgan Dennis because he is the most amazing teacher. He has taught me that miracles can be real.

I am deeply grateful for those who have supported our community over the years.

I am thankful for Gary Glazner and Marty Gerber, who believed that I could actually do this book.

Thank you to our caregivers, who are the hardest working, most loving, awesome human beings ever. You ROCK!

To all the families we have worked with over many years— your presence in our lives is an honor.

I am grateful for all the stories that have yet to be told. These stories and the people who live them will someday heal dementia and end Alzheimer's. These stories and the people living them will change all of our lives.

Mostly, I am grateful for the presence our elders have had in our lives. The toughness, humor, bravery, kindness, honesty, and creativity that these incredible human beings show on a daily basis always surprises me, and always shows me how much I still have to learn.

Prologue

Small stories

A mother and daughter hold hands, touching their foreheads together. Mom has not spoken in two years. They remain like this for several minutes, just touching foreheads, each smiling. The daughter begins to giggle. Mom laughs loudly and wraps her arms around her daughter. Mom, quietly and in a garbled voice, says, "Love you."

A woman looks at a caregiver, grabs hold of her hand and, with tears in her eyes, says, "I have Alzheimer's, don't I?" The caregiver, taken by surprise, hugs her and responds, "Yes, si. You will be okay." The woman looks around, seeming lost. Then she sits next to a much older woman and tells the caregiver, "I will help her then." In a few minutes she is helping the older woman hold her juice, and both are smiling.

It is Christmas Eve, 1975. A couple and their two young children are in a hospital room in Missouri. She is thin, sleeping fitfully. She had surgery the day before for the fourth time; this would be the last time. The man sits in a chair next to her, stroking her very short hair. The children have stopped playing and are finally quiet. The boy has Down syndrome. His red-brown hair needs a trim. He sleeps curled up on a big denim beanbag, holding a purple pig stuffed animal that is almost as big as he is. The girl lies next to her brother, books on the floor beside her. She pretends to sleep. The man begins to sing quietly, off key: "Amazing grace, how sweet the sound. . . Spirit I adore you, lay my life before you, how I love you. . . ." It is snowing. The woman takes the man's hand, and the girl falls asleep.

Small miracles like these happen every minute of every day. Choices make all of them possible: A daughter makes the choice to just be with Mom where she is. A mother makes the choice to laugh in the face of dying. A caregiver makes the choice to be honest to a client in pain and to express love at the same time. A woman makes the choice—conscious or not—to face being terminally ill by helping another. On that Christmas Eve, a mother and wife who loves her life and family chooses to fight for both even though she is so, so tired. A floor nurse, stuck working a holiday, makes the choice to disregard hospital policy and allow a family to be together. A man makes the choice to hold his family together, no matter what.

All of these people make the choice to love. This love is fierce, it is honest, it protects, and it takes risks. This love is also gentle, kind, spiritual, and funny. This love is the stuff that creates both small and large miracles. This fierce love does not hide from pain but walks into it with eyes wide open. This love ultimately wins.

Fierce Love

Fierce love, a definition

This is a book of love stories—not the heart-fluttering, romantic kind of love stories, but something else. Although love in the giving and receiving of care can indeed be tender, kind, and often sweet, giving and receiving care also includes struggle, fatigue, and even anger. Denial is also a part of the process, which can be dangerous. Emergency rooms all over this country deal with the results of denial every day. Individuals and families who run out of options end up with the uncomfortable choice of giving up, allowing care to consume them. Or they can decide to fight bad systems and, in the process, create new ways of supporting care.

This book is not about giving up. This book is also not about allowing care to become so consuming that it swallows both people—the giver and the receiver—in the process. It is about how to find, recognize, and help nurture good systems of care. In the connection of receiving and giving care, there must be balance. Both the person who needs care and the person giving care need freedom; they each need to be connected to something outside of each other.

As a caregiver myself, I am challenged daily to pay attention, not just to my brother, but also to myself. Where is my energy? Is this a healthy way to live? Part of caring for someone in our culture, maybe in all cultures, is having the energy, health, and strength to work for—and often fight for—positive change. That won't happen if we allow ourselves to believe we can do this alone. No one can do it alone, at least not in a healthy, sane way that allows both the caregiver and the person facing the stress and challenge of needing help to have full lives.

This is where the other characters in these love stories come in. Families and individuals facing the scary idea that they need help aren't the only people who struggle with the needs, boundaries, dysfunctional systems, fatigue, and frustrations that come with caregiving or needing care. The "professionals" are the other characters in the complex stories of caregiving. This group includes doctors, emergency room staff, teachers, therapists, social workers, counselors, pastors, police officers, home health aides, CNAs, direct caregiving staff, and more. Pick up any newspaper or scan the internet and you will find stories about what can happen when these people make a mistake. These professionals can be held up as heroes, which many often are. But they all struggle with the work they do and the people they serve. Often it is in this struggle where the potential for growth, connection, and love reside.

Struggle is where the word "fierce" comes in. Fierce is the ability to fight, to go beyond, to hold one's emotions at bay, and to work for the good of another. Struggle is the newly divorced young mother with a baby in a sling and a father clutching her hand, wandering the grocery store at 6:30 on a Friday night just before a holiday.

Struggle is the caregiver holding back her tears as she brings tea and cookies to the family sitting with Dad. The man has always reminded her of her own father. She sings softly to him in Spanish and hugs the grown children. The man's breathing changes, then stops.

Struggle is the EMT on his last call of the night who picks up the lady wandering the highway in her nightgown, barefoot, on a snowy January night. She is confused, yelling, cursing. He talks, flirts a bit. She relaxes, holds his hand, and won't let go. He sits with her for hours after his shift until her family can be reached.

Struggle is a retired therapist who knows she has Alzheimer's and reaches out to other people who are struggling, forcing herself to find the words to say that she needs more sleep and is always frightened. Her words help everyone she talks to.

Struggle is the sister who trades a cozy retirement for caring for her brother and becoming a constant fighter for developmental disability services. She has spent the last twelve years arguing, cajoling, and annoying the state through two different governors and political parties.

Struggle is good. It is in struggle that the best, most decent, most honorable parts of us come to light. Struggle is fierce. It takes time and energy.

All of these people show ferocity. They possess a strength that comes from within, a willingness to comfort, protect, and fight on the behalf of others. But with this strength there are always background questions: Who is there for them? From where can they draw strength? How do we work together to make these lives better?

Maybe the answers to these questions need to start by being honest about care, caregiving, and the need for care.

Numbers matter—you are not alone

Truth number one is this: Almost everyone out there at some point will either need care or will be required to care for another. According to the same joint study mentioned above from The National Alliance for Caregiving and AARP, approximately 22.3 percent of all Americans are caregivers in some capacity. This means two very important things: One, if you are a caregiver, *no matter how it feels, you are not alone*; and two, for the few of those who are not faced with either needing care or giving care at the moment, *this is not someone else's problem*.

Those caregivers out there and the people they are working so hard to care for affect the entire fabric of our society.

Truth number two is this: *You can't do this alone. No one can.* We have this fantasy that independence is how we should all measure our worth. But the fact of needing and giving care should teach all of us that none of us is fully independent. Often the effort to pretend to have independence or to hang on to independence produces results that can be dangerous, unhealthy, and expensive. The false belief that asking for help makes one weak, needy, lazy, or worthless is not only untrue, but can be expensive, dangerous, and sometimes fatal.

Families who seek out and receive help with caregiving early on have fewer emergency room visits, are able to care for their loved one longer at home, and benefit from less restrictive levels of care, such as day programs or assisted living, which are both less expensive than nursing-home care. According to several studies, the individual who receives care has a social life outside of the caregiver, and also benefits from having caregivers with lower rates of depression and chronic illness.

A few years ago, I planned a weekend trip to go hiking with an old friend of mine. I asked my brother, Morgan, if he wanted to join us. To my surprise, and I have to admit I was slightly offended at the time, he chose to stay with his caregiver, Lucy. Going to the woods with me and my boring friend was far less interesting than watching movies, going bowling, and hanging out at the mall with Lucy and her daughter. Morgan had a wonderful weekend. (Me, not so much.)

A similar story happened with one of our elders and her daughter. The elder had recently moved in to Vista. Her daughter visited daily despite having an infant, two other young children, and a taxing job. She was worried her mom would be lonely without her. During one visit, her mom's new friend walked by and Mom promptly joined her, leaving her daughter sitting alone. The daughter was then able to allow herself not to visit daily. Visiting her Mom became a treat instead of a penance. There is a time for all of us as caregivers to understand that we are not the center of the universe, and that really is a good thing.

Sadly, many people wait until care becomes more physically and medically demanding only to face long waitlists for assistance or placement. It also means that the person they are caring for will have fewer internal resources to adjust to other caregivers or make friends. One of the most important and difficult parts of being a caregiver is being unflinchingly honest about what you can and cannot do. This is complicated; not only does it require realism and the willingness to see where help is needed, but it also requires the tenacity and resolve to both access and accept help.

Families need more options and the ability to utilize those options sooner. Families also need to start looking for options before they need them. Advocacy and creating options do not help if they aren't used. Studies by the Alzheimer's Association, AARP, the National Alliance for Caregiving, and the Centers for Disease Control all show the same results: Many, many caregivers do not reach out for help or wait too long to reach out. According to AARP, less than 50 percent seek out respite care, only 28 percent seek financial assistance to aid in caregiving, and 30.3 percent die before the person they are caring for. For many of us who work in long-term care settings, this is a story we see repeated far too often, a story that needs to end.

Wonderful work is being done out there. Groups such as the Alzheimer's Association, Eden Alternative, AARP, and others provide online information and other services. Organized support groups that meet both in person and online offer information, moral support, and a safe place to share feelings. Many facilities, arts organizations, healthcare programs, veterans programs, churches, synagogues, and spiritual communities provide day programs and respite services. We do need improved access to respite in rural areas, especially in New Mexico, but many are working to improve those options. And residential care can be a loving, social, and positive experience.

Our staff and other likeminded professionals work daily to provide excellent care and to end the stereotype of the abandoned, ignored elder in facility living. The stereotypes are not helpful for families. I often wonder if all the lawyer ads looking to sue nursing homes and the news stories on care facilities that make dangerous, neglectful mistakes do more harm than good. Yes, there are bad situations. I wish there weren't. But the public fear that is based on the stereotypes all too often creates more stress on caregivers who really need to reach out for help. This can create unsafe situations as well.

A burned out caregiver is a danger to themselves and to the person in their care. I encourage people to look before they are desperate, to visit places and ask questions. In a wonderful Alzheimer's caregiver guide, Dr. Ruth Westheimer makes the point over and over to "gather information before you are at wit's end." This is good, sensible advice. Desperation allows for guilt, fear, and frustration to be the decision-makers instead of weighing pros and cons in a loving, positive way. While I have seen people over the years who were able to find just the right care by walking in from the emergency room, that is not always the case. Many people find the opposite, that procrastinating reduces the options for both elders and families.

A daughter who faced her mother's Alzheimer's disease told me that her life and her mother's life both improved when she realized that her mother's care was a marathon and not a sprint. The daughter had been a tri-athlete and trainer for many years. She likened her mother's care to preparing for a race—it was a process that took time and planning. Looking at the life she and her sister shared with their mom in this way helped all of them. By looking at options, discussing possibilities, and coordinating care together, they were able to help Mom live a fulfilling life at Vista Living Care. Both Mom and daughters were able to have lives that they could share and still have independence as well.

Burnout hurts everyone

In doing research for this book, I came across some rather disheartening statistics from the U.S. Department of Labor. Three professions—police officers, direct caregiving staff, and teachers—were listed in the top ten both for increasing demand for workers and for wages that are failing to keep up with the rate of inflation. This speaks volumes about the priority of care in our society as well as the rapidly increasing demand for care. These professions deal with people who are vulnerable, people who need help; they are based on putting others' needs first. All are based on fierce love and the motivation to protect others, to make a better future for our children, and to care for our elders. These are people who care for our past, present, and future. We all need people in these professions to be healthy, rested, and focused.

In these professions, burnout can lead to mistakes that have the potential to seriously impact the lives of others. The issue of burnout is striking for both professional and family caregivers. In her book *Burnout: The Cost of Caring*, Christina Maslach looks at the way systems disrespect professional caregivers and how this contributes to burnout. She demonstrates that a systemic lack of respect for individual caregivers (in her book, police officers, social workers, and teachers) stifles creativity and disconnects caregivers from seeing the people they care for as individual human beings. Creativity and the ability to maintain a loving human connection are the best defenses against burnout. This is true for both families and professionals. When someone you love becomes a disease first and a person second, it is not safe for either you or the person in your care.

Bill Thomas, M.D., calls loneliness, helplessness, and boredom "plagues" in his book *What Are Old People For? How Elders Will Save the World*. His work through Eden Alternative seeks to rid elders of these plagues. But in reality, burnout is a caregiver falling victim to these same plagues. If you hold up the list of dementia symptoms next to the list of burnout symptoms, you will see some striking similarities:

Dementia Symptoms	Caregiver Burnout Symptoms
• Emotional changes, such as increased anger, anxiety, depression, or agitation	• Emotional difficulties, such as anger, depression, frustration, anxiety
• Social withdrawal	• Social isolation
• Increased fatigue and disrupted sleep	• Change in sleeping habits, disrupted sleep
• Change in eating habits	• Change in eating habits
• Disorientation	• Disorientation or brain fog
• Confusion	• Decreased interest in exercise, hobbies, work etc.
• Decreased interest in exercise, hobbies, work, etc.	• Decreased immune response
• Memory loss	• Becoming family enabler or martyr
• Decreased motor function	• Decline in overall health
• Incontinence	• Irritability
• Disinhibition; sexual or socially inappropriate behavior	• Increased risk for dementia
• Cognitive decline	
• Other physical issues as the disease progresses	

To be lonely is to be unloved, to not receive love, tending, or respect for the person you are. To be bored is to be tired, to lose touch with the creative, soul-filling love of life. This comes from having no time outside of giving care, and is a result of helplessness.

Too often, caregivers, both professional and family, are left with limited options. They are saddled with systems that don't allow space for creativity and seem to be made to encourage failure. Caregivers know, in very practical ways, what they need to provide good care: day programs that are open until the workday is over, with enough staff to do the job; respite; options to pay for care without either having to use services that aren't needed or drowning in paperwork; and not having to prove that someone has dementia every few months. In short, enough common sense to be able to provide good care and still have a life.

Caregiving as a personal challenge

We need to value both the people who need care and the people who provide care. It is strange to begin writing this book in 2016, an election year. Every day on the news, whether the leaning is right or left, the idea of care and caregivers gets avoided, romanticized, diminished, or used as a punching bag. We see stories about failure, blame, and attempts to reduce human experience to tax breaks, arguing points, stereotypes, and denial, always with the push to take sides. Neither side gets to the day-to-day needs, struggles, and dreams of families, friends, spouses, and individuals. Like the lawyer ads on TV, our politics seek to assign blame without understanding the complex—and sometimes flawed—human beings whose lives are the story of caregiving.

The fact is that the need for care and the giving of care are core expressions of what it is to be human. Relationships can't be reduced to any one set of ideas or approaches. The need for care is more than a problem, a cause of stress, or a statistic. Caregiving is a challenge to see what we really are: How strong can we be? How loving? How honest? Can we see the innate value in all people? Are we capable of facing the struggle in a fierce way? Can we love and give freedom, respect, and space all at once? Do we have the courage?

Many families do not work in systems that function well. That must change. These families are constantly pulled between the needs of the person they are caring for and the money they need to earn. Companies both large and small could benefit from addressing the needs of family caregivers in ways that combine creativity, compassion, and common sense.

Decision-making—the "G words"

How do caregivers make decisions? How do caregivers find a clear, honest, and loving vision of the needs of the people they care for? How does someone who needs care have freedom and independence? How does a family in the midst of a life-ending illness find what they need to function? How do people deal with the feelings that surround losing someone they love in an often slow, painful way? Is there any way to know if we are making the right decisions for the ones we love?

The way I have been thinking about decisions lately has been to look at a set of seven words that start with the letter **G**:

Guilt can be both a motivator and an obstacle.

Grief is often deep, complicated, and long-term; like guilt, it can control decisions.

Grit is the ability to be honest, to fight for what is needed.

Gravity is the weight of care, the slow, steady, addition of loss and fatigue; gravity is also the deepening of life that comes from the care of someone in a loving, committed way.

Gratitude is the giving of and the ability to accept thanks.

Giggles is an expression of the need to share humor, joy, and the fact that parts of this journey really are funny; laughter can save a caregiver's life.

Grace is the many blessings expressed in caregiving and the ability to see them; grace is faith in life.

Ultimately there is only one decision that matters, the decision to stand by someone you love no matter where the process leads. There is no one right way to do this. Instead there is a constantly changing mosaic of decisions, acceptances, choices, a few failed attempts, and love.

Loving advice to caregivers

If you are a family caregiver working in a situation that does not embody these values, first, speak up. Second, hang in there. Be creative about how you use your time and in coming up with ideas that may allow you to be both productive with your work and care for your loved one. Stand up for the rights and needs of both the person you care for and yourself. Compromise when appropriate. Figure out what you need and what you can let go of. Be honest with yourself. Reach out for help before you need it. This applies to both work situations and services applications for the person you are caring for. Accept help when it is offered.

Like all parts of caregiving, the issues that surround work, time, finances, and funding for care all take planning. Dealing with these issues will take time. Don't wait until you are desperate or there is a crisis. My business partner, Velma, has observed that most families only start looking for help after they have been struggling for six months or more; numerous studies tend to support this observation. It will take time to get all the pieces of life balanced out. You will face waitlists, paperwork, scheduling, meetings, and more paperwork. These are part of the process. Then things will change. Keep going.

Ask lots of questions. Be annoying at times. Learn as much as possible about the disease process your loved one is facing because knowledge really is power. Forget the disease as often as possible, and face the person you love as a person. Pablo Picasso once said he learned to draw so he could let go of everything he learned. Learning about dementia is like that—know what you are facing, and then find a way to let go and get beyond the disease. Music, handholding, laughter, and rest are good places to start. I know the last thing many us feel we have time or energy for is to advocate for change and be active, but we must do it anyway because in the long run it helps. Talk about how you feel. Support others. Say thank you often. Sleep well. Eat well. Exercise whenever possible. This one is tough, but it has to happen: Find time away from caregiving. Give the person you care for some space of their own as well. They tire of us too.

Love fiercely.

Dementia 101: Facing Facts—and Getting Beyond Them

Getting beyond "Alzheimer's sucks"

"Ruth, some things just suck." In 1999, an oncologist said this to me before I started the chemotherapy that would help me beat cancer. Those words helped me. They came with a deeply honest, compassionate discussion of the help that I needed and the fact that even though I did not have insurance or money at the time, I had one choice to make: Fight and live or wait and die. I would spend more than a year fighting and more than ten years dealing with the financial issues around this. It was worth it. I love my life. The time with my brother, the work I have done, the people I have loved, and all the painting and gardening would not have happened without my facing the "sucks" part. Honesty kept me alive.

So why does this story end up in a book about dementia and caregiving?

A T-shirt I got from a caregiver conference actually reads, "Alzheimer's sucks." The truth is, any progressive dementia sucks. This is not a cynical, hopeless, or jaded statement. It is simply true. This process is tough and, currently, ultimately fatal for the person facing it. It is a struggle for everyone who loves the person. There will be tears and anger, there will be fatigue, and there is no cure. However, there is still life in the process: love, joy, and yes, hope. Hope in the face of death. Joy in the face of sheer terror. Love in the deepest, toughest, rawest, purest form. Yes, this disease sucks. Now it is time face it and move beyond it.

Facts and knowledge are frightening. They are also powerful. Knowing the process that you or someone you love is going through is freeing in many ways. Realistic expectations are useful in preparing for the future. That does not mean giving up; it means being proactive early on. Knowing as much as possible about what is ahead allows individuals and families to better manage resources, enlist emotional support, and have more choices. Unpredictability can be part of certain dementia processes (Lewy body disease, in particular), but understanding the basic process helps make this less frightening. Being aware of what is going on in the brain and the body can help create patience for oneself and others. Knowledge is a way to pull back from the emotions that can swallow anyone facing a life threatening illness. This does not mean to discount feelings; it means to express them in a productive way.

Proactive knowledge is useful in many ways. For example, according to a 2016 study by UC Irvine, between 5 and 15 percent of all dementias can be reversed or stabilized with a strict protocol. (However, the results are mixed.) Certain conditions such as hypothyroidism, B12 deficiency, addictions, and untreated depression or PTSD all may present symptoms that mimic dementia. If you live in an area where Lyme disease is present and memory problems seem to be accompanied by joint pain and fatigue, get tested. Patricia Gerbarg, M.D., has written on the ability of Lyme disease to create a pseudo dementia. Treatment for these issues, if timely and effective, can return someone to normal functioning. The word "timely" is very important here. If memory and judgment issues are getting in the way of daily life, one should see a doctor and get a thorough workup.

Person, place, or thing?

Before I began working with dementia, I worked with addictions treatment. Something we were frequently told to look for was "person, place, or thing." "Person" meant relationships with family, friends, and co-workers. "Place" was applied to someone's ability or inability to maintain a home and pay the rent or mortgage. "Thing" involved the ability to manage finances and make healthy choices around money and spending. Looking at person, place, or thing meant asking the question, Was drinking or doing drugs affecting any of these areas in a negative way? If so, there was a problem, and someone needed help.

This concept can apply to memory and cognitive impairment as well. Problems in any of these areas are a signal that what is happening is not a normal response to aging. While we all have different ways of keeping house or balancing a checkbook, if someone is struggling with a skill they were once good at, there is an issue. Families should not wait for a crisis to seek the advice of a doctor or to begin helping an elderly family member with "person, place, or thing." That delay could be fatal.

Executive functioning

Many of the progressive dementias affect what is called "executive functioning" as well as short-term memory. Diseases like Alzheimer's, Lewy body disease, and frontotemporal dementia change a person's ability to function in the world. These disease processes all have detrimental effects on the frontal and temporal lobes of the brain, which control executive functioning. Tasks that require decision-making, planning, reasoning, tracking, or judgment will become increasingly difficult to complete. Executive functioning is the ability to organize one's day—to buy groceries, pay bills, etc. It includes all the basic and not-so-basic tasks we need to track in order to survive. It also controls the ability to discern and respond in emergency situations.

Having a strong and aware support system early on that allows freedom and at the same time provides a safe haven for an elder is crucial. But this can be difficult because of another skill that is part of executive functioning—the ability to recognize when there is a problem. Self-awareness is also a function of the frontal and temporal lobes. Thus, denial and covering up are frequently part of the disease process.

Denial

While the illnesses that create progressive dementia are not contagious, some of the problems an individual who has dementia may face can be "caught" by the caregiver. Denial is one of these problems. One of the statements I have heard over and over in my work at Vista Living Care is that one's mother, father, husband, wife, or friend "is not like those people." These may be the most dangerous and, in some ways, the most unloving words in the English language. No one with dementia is like any other person with dementia. To use Velma's words, everyone is a snowflake. But just like every snowflake needs certain weather conditions to form, everyone with dementia needs help in some part of their lives, and often in their own special way.

Denial interferes with the ability to get the right help at the right time. First, it decreases the chances of getting timely and effective treatment for the percentage of dementias that is either curable or not progressive. Denial also cuts into the ability of families to access care and financial resources, and to create living environments that are both nurturing and secure. Denial can prevent medication from being used in a positive way. (Medications for progressive dementias are often more effective when started in the mild to moderate stages.) Depression,

PTSD, and addictions all have the potential to open the door to progressive dementia. Certain frontotemporal lobe dementias can create addictive behaviors in someone who has not previously shown these issues, which will in turn accelerate the dementia. The relationship that each of these issues has with cognitive functioning is very complex. Despite this complexity, early treatment produces better outcomes.

Treatment is not only about medications. Dr. Robert Levine, in his book *Defying Dementia: Understanding and Preventing Alzheimer's and Related Disorders*, writes that counseling, exercise, good nutrition, and pursuing creative and educational outlets have been shown to reduce the risk for early- to middle-stage dementia and can help make the process more bearable. Creative therapies are also very comforting in all stages by offering individuals an outlet for self-expression, the pleasure of creating, and the opportunity to explore new roles later in life. An open and loving approach brings security and comfort to elders in all stages of the disease; realistic expectations innately create comfort.

Facing dementia head on without stigma or judgment allows individuals and families to create a means of caregiving that can allow for a life lived in a positive, resilient way. Hiding symptoms, not discussing problems, and not reaching out for help do just the opposite. Dr. Richard Taylor was a psychotherapist whose writing, lectures, and deep honesty about his own experience of living with Alzheimer's have deeply affected how dementia care is thought of throughout the world. Much of his work was about two topics: the profound stigma of dementia, and the idea that despite a diagnosis of dementia, a person still lives and can engage in life. Denial of the process comes directly out of the stigma that this amazing man spoke of with such intense awareness.

Denial is also cynical; it denies the life people have within them despite the struggle of this disease process. Denial decreases access to creative, healing outlets and limits the choices that someone will have for the future. Another saying that comes from addiction treatment but is also true for facing dementia is, "You are only as sick as your secrets."

The healing power of honesty

Several years ago, the daughter of one of our elderly ladies allowed a reporter from our local newspaper, *The Santa Fe New Mexican,* to photograph her mother throughout a week of her daily life. Her mother was heading into the later stages of Alzheimer's disease. While she was still a vibrant woman, she was living with profound physical and emotional struggles. Her daughter struggled with accepting her mother's changes but decided to do the project anyway, openly discussing Mom's illness and her own fears, grief, and joy. This was an act of courage.

The result of this honest collaboration was an article that was both difficult and deeply healing for the daughter. The open discussion of the process her mother was facing helped the daughter cope with making decisions for her mom. The article also helped push our state to sign the Silver Alert into law, creating a registry program (by city or county, depending on the area) for seniors modeled on the highly successful Amber Alert. This tracking system has saved lives. Her mother relished the idea of being in the paper and helping her community. By openly sharing the "sucks" part of Alzheimer's disease, a family, a community, and a state benefitted and began to take proactive steps in making life better for elders.

Ecosystem of dementia

Dementia is basically a cluster of symptoms. According to several sources, these include:
- Emotional changes, such as increased anger, anxiety, depression, or agitation

- Social withdrawal
- Increased fatigue and disrupted sleep
- Change in eating habits
- Disorientation
- Confusion
- Decreased interest in exercise, hobbies, work, etc.
- Memory loss
- Decreased motor function
- Incontinence
- Disinhibition; sexual or socially inappropriate behavior
- Cognitive decline
- Other physical issues as the disease progresses

We used to refer to dementia as an umbrella, with the rain-drops falling off it representing different diseases. Now, I would change that image to a tree with many branches coming off the same trunk. The trunk is the basic set of symptoms; the branches are different diseases. All of the many variations, sub-groups, and responses to the disease processes become the leaves. The root system would be the many causes and factors that are far from being fully understood.

But that tree is not a separate entity. Like the stands of aspen in the mountains around Santa Fe, the individual trees share a common root system. Caregivers are part of that shared root system. If we keep going with this idea, the soil, rocks, and water are all of us. This greater community can provide refuge or make life harder for elders and caregivers. As a society, we have to decide which kind of soil we will create.

Eden Alternative talks about care as tending a garden. I love this image, but my experience as a caregiver has been more tangled, wilder, and harder to control. The aspens feel that way to me. Those aspens, like the families, elders, and caregivers I have known, are part of an amazing, and often complex, ecosystem of care. Like those aspens, they are beautiful, tough, and deeply connected to one another.

Definitive diagnosis? Or is it just too complicated?

Is it really important to know which type of dementia someone is facing? The answer, like many other parts of this process, is quite gray. No, yes, sometimes, maybe...even with highly invasive testing, the only exact way to diagnose is through autopsy. The level of testing needs to be put to the question of quality of life: Will it help elders feel more comfortable or safe, or allow them to be in an environment that makes them happy?

In simple terms, diagnosis is a ruling-out process. Testing is done, observations are made, and the puzzle pieces are put into place. This is why having a good medical workup is important. This workup can test for and get treatment started for any issues that can be fixed or stabilized. But the puzzle pieces that seem to come together early on do not always stay the same; it is complicated, and it is progressive. Though from a layperson's point of view it may seem like guesswork, it is closely considered and well thought out. Follow-up and having an open, honest dialogue are important. It is crucial to work with a doctor who will *listen* to caregivers and elders.

As the process goes on, this can make a huge difference in the quality of life for everyone involved. While the beginning and end of most progressive dementias are similar, there can be differences in how certain diseases progress in the middle stages. Different disease processes will change how medication affects people, and can also cause physical changes that may become severe and decrease life expectancy. It is important to have a basic framework to understand the changes that an individual will likely face. Simply knowing that certain people with Lewy body dementia may hallucinate or can fluctuate rapidly in terms of mental clarity or behavior can allow for better care. Understanding that some people with frontotemporal lobe dementia might develop the drive to eat nonfood items can allow better home safety. If a diagnosis can be made in a way that is not invasive or uncomfortable, it can lead to better and more useful guesswork, which can lead to better care and more comfort. Getting help is important. Professional care-givers may be better suited to dealing with certain scenarios.

For many elders who face dementia, and really for anyone in the midst of a life-ending illness, there is a point where medical testing and treatment simply become more uncomfortable, invasive, and stressful than helpful. According to the Eden Alternative, "Medical treatment should be the servant of genuine human caring, not its master."

What it is

Alzheimer's disease, first discovered in 1906 by Dr. Alois Alzheimer, is the most researched of the progressive dementias. According to the Alzheimer's Association, this disease accounts for between 60 and 80 percent of all progressive dementias. (These numbers are debated as more research is done and the ways of diagnosing become more precise.) Currently, Alzheimer's diagnoses have only one division: If the onset occurs before age sixty-five, it is considered "early onset Alzheimer's disease"; after age sixty-five, it is simply "Alzheimer's disease."

Age is the most definitive predictor of Alzheimer's. After age sixty, the risk doubles with every ten years of age. By ninety, one has a 50 percent chance of being diagnosed with Alzheimer's disease.

Early onset Alzheimer's is more likely to have a genetic com-ponent than later onset, and it seems to progress at a different rate, though this is still a subject of debate. In 2016, 60 *Minutes* did an excellent feature on a community in Antioquia, Colom-bia, which has the largest concentration of families on the planet who carry a rare genetic mutation of the fourteenth chromosome. (People with a defect on this chromosome con-sistently develop early onset Alzheimer's disease.) Long-term study and medication testing are being conducted to search for a way to interrupt the cascade process of dementia and to improve the chances for someone with this defective chromosome to not contract Alzheimer's disease. The work is a positive step in the search for a vaccine.

According to other current research, the most clear-cut genetic link to Alzheimer's disease is Down syndrome. The amyloid precursor protein, or APP, which triggers the production of plaques in the brain, is located on the twenty-first chromosome. In Down syndrome, this chromosome is replicated. This causes an overexpression of APP in the brain tissue, increasing the risk for Alzheimer's disease. Due to the natural tendency for someone with Down syndrome to age more rapidly, people with Down syndrome may show signs of Alzheimer's as young as forty.

Alzheimer's disease is characterized by short-term memory loss that grows more profound over the years. Short-term memory loss gradually becomes deep memory loss, increased confusion, and changes in temperament; physical changes in balance, walking ability, and incontinence will also occur for many elders. Elders often express repetitive questions or behaviors. All of these changes lead to a decreased ability to function.

There is a beautiful line in a book by the French author Collette: "It was merely physical, which means it shook the soul." This statement is true of Alzheimer's disease: The changes in the brain are physical. The effects of those changes shake the souls of the elder as well as the souls of his or her loved ones. The physical changes in the brain that create these problems involve the formation of amyloid plaques and tau protein tangles. These tangles in turn block neuronal connections, causing a cascade of neuron death. This causes the brain to shrink. Each individual facing this illness will respond to the changes in the brain in their own way. But it is important to remember that *the person is still in there*. This is something that all involved need to remind themselves of each day.

Snowflakes, changes, and stages

My experience working with people facing Alzheimer's disease and other progressive dementias has taught me that while there are common struggles in the process, each person will have areas of strength and of weakness. The most common tool for assessing the level of the disease process is Dr. Barry Reisberg's Global Deterioration Scale. I find it a useful tool to help families who have difficulty facing what their loved one is going through; it can be a needed dose of realism at times. Ignoring the "sucks" part of Alzheimer's can create discomfort. The Global Deterioration Scale is focused on the "sucks" parts of the disease. It defines the entire process by the loss of skills and increase of symptoms.

That said, most people do not progress in neat, clear-cut ways. Elders can plateau or change rapidly during different stages of the disease process. This can be extremely disorienting for caregivers as well as for the person facing the disease. Most will excel at certain areas of their lives and struggle with—or be completely unable to perform—other tasks. Verbal ability is one area on which functioning is measured, but this can be deceptive. We worked for several years with a gentleman who could astutely discuss current politics and *New York Times* articles and could tell you a daily schedule if you asked. The schedule was largely fiction, but he recited it in a clear, concise, and convincing manner. His doctor bought it. However, the same man could not get dressed, brush his teeth, or take medications without considerable hands-on help. He had extreme difficulty with sequencing. He simply could not remember that the socks went on before the shoes or that toothpaste went on the toothbrush and not the comb. No notes, occupational therapy, or modeling could restore his ability to do a series of tasks in a specific order. That part of his brain simply did not work. It did not make him any less articulate or intelligent; it just meant he needed help in certain parts of his life.

Right now, I am working with a lady who is completely non-verbal. She is also very calm, gracious, and self-contained. She has held onto the ability to calm herself and resolve her emotions. One of her peers has excellent verbal abilities and is highly creative but is unable to manage her emotions. She also has increasing difficulties processing day-to-day stimulation and frequently becomes overwhelmed. Both are in the middle to late stages of dementia, and both face serious challenges every day. But they also have strengths that allow them some freedom from the disease.

These stories come back to the snowflake idea. Each person who faces Alzheimer's is not only a unique individual, but they are facing a process that will manifest in their lives in very particular ways. That said, each of these unique individuals will need some help with basic parts of their lives. Without this help, they will not function.

Repeat, and repeat again

Repetitive questions, statements, and actions are probably the most well-known feature of dementia, the stereotype of Alzheimer's disease. Imagine what it really means to lose short-term memory. It is not that the person with progressive dementia forgets an event or something they were told; to them, it never happened. There was no event, or phone call, or lunch, or whatever else. The brain never recorded it. Velma asks, "We don't ask a blind person to see; why do we ask someone with Alzheimer's to remember?"

I think I know the answer to this question. It has to do with the fact that many people with dementia display paradoxes in the ways they function in the world. A man who can discuss politics should remember that he ate breakfast or how to go to the bathroom. Someone who seems so together should not have to ask the same question every three minutes. It seems to defy logic. But in the world of dementia, it makes perfect sense for someone to ask the same question two hundred times a day and to also remember the day they met their spouse fifty years ago with absolute clarity. The brain made that recording; it did not record breakfast.

Trying to live in that paradoxical, illogical world called dementia is why caregivers need rest. It is also why Vista Living emphasizes the importance of caregivers dwelling in the elder's reality rather than trying to drag the elder into "our" reality.

Diamonds, pearls, and elders

The "Gems Theory" is a strength-based approach developed by Teepa Snow, an occupational therapist and lead educator on dementia and care. Compassionate, gentle, and graceful, it can be helpful for caregivers because it illustrates the stages of dementia with various gemstones: Sapphire (healthy brain is "true blue" though processing is slower); Diamond (cognition is clear, but may be cutting and rigid, seeing help as a threat); Emerald ("naturally flawed" with moments of clarity mixed with periods of loss in logic and perspective); Amber (caught in a moment of time, can feel threatened by care due to differences in perspective and ability); Ruby ("deep red" masks detail—movements and transitions must be guided, skilled abilities lost); and Pearl (hidden like a pearl in an oyster shell, capabilities are minimal).

Ms. Snow has done a great service to elder care by reminding us all of the innate value of elders. She also publishes an online journal on her website that is very supportive for both professionals and families (www.teepasnow.com).

Balance and respect

My hesitation with dementia stages and scales is that we need to see both the strengths and the struggles, both the "Alzheimer's sucks" part of things and the innate humanity and resiliency in every elder's life. Balancing this has been the bulk of my work for the past twenty years.

An elder we have worked with for the past six years recently began to lose his ability to walk. After many interventions, physical therapy, medication, and neurologist visits, nothing could stop this path of the disease. In his words, "Goddamn legs don't work!" His anger was not a behavior to be medicated away; it was deep anger and grief, a part of his personhood. You don't stop being a real human being once you develop dementia. As caregivers, we must honor the whole person. This man needed to curse and talk; he needed to grieve. That has to be respected.

Just because someone needs help taking a shower or remembers in a different way does not mean that they don't contribute to society. Needing help doesn't mean life is over. Over my years of working with Alzheimer's, I have met elders who were resilient, loving, funny, creative and strong. They are artists, gardeners, dancers, fighters, teachers, friends, and people in love. They have lives. They can teach great lessons to the "normal" world. Things that come naturally to elders facing dementia are struggles the rest of the world faces, such as getting over being angry, getting past judging others, being affectionate, and being forgiving. Those of us who can remember what we had for breakfast and know how to get dressed also struggle with being kind, open-minded, and forgiving of others. Often we become cynical, burned out, and lazy. Who needs more help, really?

The Brain and the Body

As the cascade of Alzheimer's disease moves through the brain, it begins to take the body with it. Individual elders will face these challenges in different ways, but most will face these issues: Fatigue, disrupted sleep, wandering, sundowning (explained further later), incontinence, decreased tolerance of daily stimulation, and changes in eating habits, which all come from increasing damage in an elder's brain. These changes are the result of the physical death of neurons in the brain, thus beginning the process of shaking the soul.

The place where the brain and body meet in Alzheimer's is the place that changes the life of an elder and everyone who loves them. Care is no longer a distant future; it is a tangible need. Confusion creates the need for what is often demanding physical care. These changes are painful for caregivers, both family and professional. Often these developments force caregivers to make changes. For many, these hold the seeds of crisis moments.

Just tired

Increased fatigue is caused by the brain being stressed. This is not a reflection on the caregiver, facility, day program, spouse, or anyone else. "Normal" people will use about 25 percent of their calories to support brain function; under stress, that can exceed 50 percent. With Alzheimer's and other progressive dementias, the brain is under constant stress. It is stressful to simply sort out the day and one's surroundings. In addition, Alzheimer's affects the REM sleep cycle, which can interfere with cognitive functioning and increase confusion. If the person you care for naps, it doesn't mean you are boring, and it does not necessarily mean they need something to do. If they live in a residential program, they are probably not over medicated. They may simply be tired.

According to Dr. Larry Dossey, gentle, natural routines and simple, calming pleasures become very important to people with Alzheimer's and for caregivers. Consistency is helpful in improving the quality of sleep for anyone, but for someone with dementia, it can be grounding and give a structure to life that an elder cannot create without help and support. A gentle routine improves quality of sleep and life.

Disrupted sleep

Many people with Alzheimer's face another sleep issue— nighttime wakefulness, or disrupted sleep. The circadian rhythm, like everything in our lives, is directed by the brain. As brain function becomes more and more diminished, some elders have difficulty staying asleep. Disrupted sleep is one part of Alzheimer's disease and other dementias that is "contagious" for family caregivers, and it can be relentless. It is one of the main reasons for placement in assisted living and nursing homes.

At Vista Living Care, we do not use medications to get elders to a "normal" sleep cycle. They keep their own pattern. This means we do have elders who "work the night shift" and go to sleep after breakfast, or doze and watch the chickens. We have naturally gravitated to this approach and have tended to be very apprehensive about sleep medication for elders. The Eden Alternative has done extensive research on this issue and, just like their overall drug-free approach to dementia care, stresses that a pill is not a solution for many problems, including sleep disturbance. However, this approach is much tougher and less safe for home caregivers.

Though medications come with problems, this does not mean they should be completely ruled out; even the dreaded antipsychotics can at times allow for comfort and safety. But like so many other parts of this process, it's complicated. With drugs, there can be an increased risk for falls, and confusion and fatigue can increase. This end result only makes life harder for the caregiver, which in turn makes life harder for the elder. Burnout lives here.

While on call several years ago, I got an early-morning call from a woman who was crying in the emergency room, looking for a bed for her husband. The call was ended by a sudden hang-up. When I called back several times, there was no answer. A few hours later, there was another call, this time from a local professional: Could I do an emergency admission? It was one of the few times in almost eighteen years that there was a bed available.

He was a charming, handsome, and temperamental man in his seventies; his wife was the same age, beautiful in a willowy way. And she was beyond tired. He was often awake at night, angry and yelling. He had wandered away from their home several times. This time, like the other times, she followed him. But this time he did not calm down and come back to her. And this time, she was just too tired to keep going.

When he crossed a major street at around 3 a.m., she just stopped and sat down on the sidewalk in tears. She broke. The police were called, she was taken to the emergency room and hospitalized, and he was later found near their home, with no memory of the incident. When the home was checked, it was in shambles. They had both been seeing a local doctor who, in her commitment to be his advocate and encourage independence, missed how fragile the entire situation had become. I will always wonder if the wife had tried to express how tired she was, or had just kept saying, "I'm fine."

One of our caregivers adopted their cats. The local professional cleaned their house (a difficult process) and called each of their families. While at Vista, with the help of a psychiatrist, he stabilized and then moved to be closer to his sister, out of state. She moved to be closer to her children, in a different state. The marriage effectively ended.

I think of them often and wonder if things could have been different—if they had had the "some things just suck" discussion months or even years earlier, if when their families called someone had thought, We need to see them. I wonder if the smart, loving people around them got so distracted by how well-spoken, creative, and intelligent they both were and forgot to check on the groceries, or the pets, or to ask her when was the last time she'd slept. I wonder what could have been different if the people involved had really listened with their hearts and their common sense.

I find Arianna Huffington's book *The Sleep Revolution: Transforming Your Life, One Night at a Time* useful. It looks at sleep—or the lack of it—in our modern world. She refers to sleep deprivation as a "chief symptom of civilization's disease, which is burnout." Alzheimer's caregivers frequently end up working the "third shift" when caring for a loved one who is awake and wandering or rummaging at night. This is simply not sustainable.

Engaging the world—good and not-so-good stimulation

Keeping the world at bay brings us to another set of changes that elders with dementia face—a decreasing ability to process stimulation from the world around them. With dementia, the veil between the elder and the noise, visual imagery, and touch of the world is pulled away. The ability to sort out sensation diminishes. Stimulation becomes a complicated and nuanced issue.

I remember getting a call one day from a woman with questions about her father. She was talking quickly, telling me that Dad was in a "wonderful place where there were always activities" but was "acting out a lot." When I finally got a chance to respond, I asked if just maybe there might be too much activity for Dad. Before I could explain, she hung up on me.

There is a myth that more stimulation will help slow the disease process, which feeds into the guilt that caregivers often feel. The myth of constant activity speaks to the illusion we all have when someone we love is dying. There has to be a miracle out there. There has to be some way to fix this if we just do something more. If we just try one more therapy or pay for one more service, maybe the person we love will get a little better. But the facts here are quite different. Reality after dementia is different from reality before dementia. While there are ways to create comfort, to engage with life and show love, if the dementia is progressive, there is no way to make it go away. The results of this myth are simply overstimulation and exhaustion.

Good, healing stimulation is natural and respectful; noisy, demeaning busyness is exhausting. Too often, what gets passed off as "recreation programs for elders" tends to fall into the second category. I have also seen loving, well-intended families burn out their beloved elders by trying to keep them doing "what they've always done." Many elders will rise to the occasion, meaning they will expend a huge amount of energy to accomplish the task before them or to "enjoy" an activity. The family member then goes home feeling better because they have "done something," and the elder falls apart.

"Rising to the occasion" is a term in dementia care that addresses the ability of elders to pull themselves together for someone whom they feel has authority, or for someone they love. This is a very real phenomenon.

One of our elders, Millie, had been going on outings with a local dementia expert for several years. Over time, Millie developed a special friendship with this lady. They would go out for lunch and to galleries, attend events, and enjoy Santa Fe. One of their favorite lunch spots had been Souper Salad for the variety of healthy options and easy access to chocolate brownies. This restaurant is very bright and loud. As Millie got deeper into the dementia process, she became more fatigued after outings.

Early on, Millie would take a nap a after an outing and wake refreshed for a pleasant evening. But after a couple of months, she would have a hard time resting after an outing. She became increasingly angry and tearful. We also noticed changes as a whole—she would cover her ears if it were noisy, and she began struggling more with eating and getting dressed. She began to hit, bite, and kick caregivers and peers after outings. Millie was doing well during the outings, but afterward she would fall apart. We decided that our elder was rising to the occasion to impress her friend and becoming overstimulated. She stretched her abilities until she was simply exhausted. We responded by changing the type of outing to quieter venues. This worked for a while, but at some point Millie simply needed to be home. The "Souper Salad Day" had come to mean too noisy, too many choices, too tiring—too much.

In judging a healthy level of stimulation, we must remember that the changes inside the brain take energy and require an individual to concentrate more to accomplish tasks. Visual images, depth perception, startle response, and hearing all change in Alzheimer's and other dementias, and processing can be tiring. These elders also have less of a filter for noise, visual changes, and sound, so these things can easily become overwhelming. With exhaustion come confusion, risk for falls, tension, anger, poor eating, and other difficulties. This can happen even when an elder really loves the activity.

This is not to say we should avoid outings and activities, but rather to structure the time before and after with thought and care. It is important to build downtime into a major event. Even happy, loving events are stressful. We celebrate beautiful family and holiday gatherings in our Vista ecosystem. The elders enjoy these events, as do the families. Everyone dresses up, eats, dances, and enjoys great company and food. Then, for the next couple of days, the elders relax, listen to quiet music, nap, and rest. Rest is important. Naps are okay. Dementia, as it progresses, makes the world smaller and slower. We need to respect that.

All progressive dementias are by nature terminal illnesses, but the dying process is stretched into years as opposed to weeks or months. This might seem like an odd place for a note about terminal illness, but this is why I include it here: Everyone has the right, as much as possible, to live their life until it is over. However, most people's energy levels change during the dying process; they soften. This does not mean that elders should experience boredom or a lack of challenge, but the recovery time from an event such as a concert or a walk in the park increases. Elders require more rest to process and enjoy the world around them.

I appreciate this more as my brother's health has changed. For years we've had a running joke that Morgan should run for mayor because he can't go out without running into people he knows. He has spent his years in Santa Fe always on the move: going to libraries, the farmers' market, the Plaza, galleries, and every cafe in town; he even bowled with the Special Olympics. But with the fading of his heart, he has become slower, quieter, and softer. He will still dance, and he still loves seeing people and eating out, but now he needs long breaks in between. After an outing, he will go home and sleep, and the next day needs to be slow. He needs recovery time. Our elders function similarly.

Sundowning

Sundowning is a response to the changing light of approaching evening that involves increased confusion, anxiety, restlessness, sadness, and general crankiness for people with Alzheimer's. Many studies and resources offer excellent information about this and other behavioral issues, which in truth are often less about behavior and more about the loss of the ability to soothe oneself.

Our way of approaching this at Vista Living Care is to soften. When I say soften, what I mean is to become more quiet and gentle, to focus on comfort and peace. We will turn the movie off or put on a beautiful video without sound, play soft music (or none at all), offer nice food or a cup of tea, do light exercise, take a walk, or just be with someone in a gentle way. We simplify the daily routine as much as possible at this time of day, focusing only on the essential. These actions may not always work, but they have helped us.

Remember that we all need space at times, including people facing dementia. Sundowning is, in some ways, a deep body memory. It corresponds to the time of day when most of us wrap up our work, take care of children, or get stuck in traffic—all the anxiety-producing frustrations of life. It is hardwired into all of us, but dementia strips away the ability to cover or soften it. For this reason, some simplified mindfulness techniques, such as simply holding hands and taking deep breaths, can relax both elder and caregiver.

Neuroscientist V.S. Ramachandran writes extensively on the complexity of the human brain and on its innate resilience. He talks about neurobiology in terms of how deeply the body and the brain seek to function, seek to live. The deeper evolutionary meaning to sundowning is about protection and safety. For early humans, darkness was not safe, and somewhere in the neurons of our brains, we remember this. Somewhere inside the brain with dementia is a will to seek safety, to heal, to seek comfort, and to live. Our job as caregivers is to attempt to be a bridge to this place.

Wandering

Understanding the problem of wandering—the motivation for it, the danger of it, and how to approach it—is crucial in dementia care.

Elders facing dementia wander for many reasons. I see it not as a "behavior," but a coping response. Wandering is a full-body response to feelings, stressors, anxieties, or fears. Wandering can be a release of energy, a means of self-soothing. Wandering can be an escape from overwhelming noise or other stimulation. Wandering can also come from the kind of deep, evolutionary memory that sundowning is connected to. This shows up in the need to *go*, the need to get somewhere and take care of someone or something. Reasoning and explaining will not change the reality that the person with Alzheimer's is in, nor will it calm the need to *go*.

Many elders facing dementia wander in the evenings and nights. This makes sense in a disease process way, but for caregivers, it can be frightening and stressful. When encountering a wandering elder, caregivers should remember to breathe and present calm. Their fear or frustration will only increase the fear and frustration of the elder. Our job, and it is a hard job, is to reduce the stress in an elder's already stressed out, hyper-vigilant brain. We have to share calm even when we do not feel it.

Wandering can be a life or death issue in cities, but especially in rural areas. I suggest a practical approach. Start with finding out if your state has a Silver Alert; if so, sign your loved one up. Also, sign up with the MedicAlert + Alzheimer's Association's Safe Returnprogram. (See Resources and References section.) Get to know your neighbors, and be open about the fact that you are caring for someone who might lose their way.

Many studies suggest that routine physical activity that is both repetitive and meaningful can decrease the need to wander. Doing simple activities such as sweeping, gardening, raking leaves, walking the dog, or dancing can be a source of pleasure and can reduce the need to wander. Always offer water; thirst can increase both confusion and agitation, increasing the need to wander. Food, music, and pets can be positive distractions.

Frankly, caring for someone with dementia is often a matter of buying time with distractions.

We cannot reason away or explain the need to *not go*. I suggest going with the disease rather than pushing against it. Go with the person's story in a respectful way; you will not change the reality the elder lives in anyway. I worked with a lady for several years who worried every evening about picking up her children, who were in their sixties. I agreed to accept her reality that the rabbi and his wife were picking up the children and coming for dinner. So we would wipe the tables, and she would help pour the drinks. By the time the drinks were poured, she was relaxed and ready to eat supper. Somehow in helping to set the table for dinner, the children were returned to their proper place in time.

Should wandering become unsafe for your loved one or for you, residential care is not "giving up."

I work in an amazing Vista home that is "secure." The door is locked and covered by a mural of *El Santuario de Chimayo*—a celebrated church in the little town of Chimayo, about thirty miles from Santa Fe. This symbol of hope and healing is a graceful way to make the exit door vanish. The mural is also a good way to get people talking and sharing stories. (Once past that door, there is a second locked door to the outside.)

Other illusions we use include changing the color and texture of the floor to create the appearance of a hole, or a drop. In doing this we use one problem from the disease process— depth perception difficulties—to solve another problem from the disease process—wandering. (I would caution families to think long and hard before using physical changes to the environment in their own homes. Many of the ideas that are effective and graceful in assisted living would not feel the same for the caregiver in their own home.)

There is currently a debate among dementia professionals about the use of locked, or "secure," homes. Some feel this is a restraint on the freedom of elders. But is it really freedom if the obsessions and stressors of a disease control an elder's actions? We work hard to be vigilant and cautious, but our beautiful home is in a semi-rural area where wandering can create a huge risk for injury or death. New Mexico loses seniors in rural areas to exposure every year. This is one reason that the state has become proactive with the Silver Alert.

I think of our home as an intentional community. Many people attend retreats to celebrate their faith, renew their marriages, or explore their creativity. In many ways, we are a retreat. We have created a space that is both loving and safe for anyone facing dementia. We seek to be a place of refuge, a place that is both connected to the outside world and intentionally separate. That locked door is simply a marker that we are a place where elders have the freedom to be safe and respected. Their comfort decides how much of the world is allowed in and how much of the world is kept at bay.

Bathroom blues and white knuckle functioning

Incontinence and needing help with personal hygiene do not happen overnight. Most people fade into them. Mishaps occur, anxiety increases, and minor disarray becomes more and more prevalent until it grows into major disarray. Some elders will obsess over needing a bathroom (the nervous pees) or obsess about getting ready, often starting hours earlier and still not being ready for the day at noon.

Resistance is often strongest as someone is beginning to need help. In addictions work, the term "white knuckle sobriety" refers to someone who is just barely hanging on, fighting just to function that day, and the next. In dementia there is "white knuckle functioning" when an elder fights each day to hold on to a skill or a way of living, sometimes to satisfy a spouse or a family member. Independence is held on to in an often painful way. But anything that is held onto in a white knuckle way exacts a cost. Anger, fear, sadness, and stress are the emotional costs. Disheveled clothes, broken pipes, unpaid bills, kidney infections—and disappearing—are some of the physical costs.

There is actually an odd bit of good news to all of this. Most elders ultimately adjust or relax into having someone help them and are then free to explore better things than fighting to hold on to some everyday skill. Suddenly their mental energy is free to be affectionate, to be creative, to love a pet, to have a life that has meaning. Getting there is often hard and there will be struggle, but it is possible to need lots of hands-on help and still live a good life. We see this frequently at Vista. An elder moves in, adjusts to accepting help, and then lets go of the white-knuckle way of living. They relax into who they truly are beneath the fight to "hold it together." The paradox is that in many ways, they become more independent, more engaged in life around them. The fight to keep up the illusion of independence ends, and the person finds more freedom.

Teeth are another piece of the hygiene puzzle. With the understanding of how invasive this must feel, we encourage as much independence as possible, give help when needed, and encourage families to increase dental cleanings to every three months. There is no perfect answer here—find a realistic dentist. Brushing or flossing three times a day would be a form of torture for someone with middle- to late-stage Alzheimer's. Try having your own partner brush or floss your teeth and see if you're not ready for a divorce.

I work with an awesome caregiver who has been with us for more than a decade. When she started her job, she was an attractive twenty-three-year-old. She was helping a gentleman who had a tendency to be stubborn throughout his life; he also had a tendency to enjoy the company of women. She became his "teeth whisperer," mostly because he seemed to appreciate holding her hand and checking her out. She was happy that he had great teeth. It was a positive relationship, though on her part it might have been a bit clueless. It was also rare. But it did prove that occasionally, people can enjoy getting their teeth brushed by someone else.

Shadowing

Shadowing, when a person with dementia tries to keep a caregiver within sight at all times, is part of Alzheimer's and other progressive dementias. While it is more emotional than physical, shadowing shares one thing with the struggles of incontinence and hygiene: It is relentless. Shadowing is part of the deepest waters of progressive dementia. It is a soul pain for both elder and caregiver. It is one person desperately searching for safety, holding on to life, and another person who is often too exhausted to give anything more.

Someone with any progressive dementia lacks short-term memory. Thus, when they don't see someone, that person has been gone "forever." Elders will often say to a devoted family member, "I never see you." The guilt, pain, and frustration that result from hearing this are mind-bending. But this is not about the family member; it is about how misperceptions of time cross with human instinct and the fight for life. Often, the caregiver becomes the only touchstone an elder has in a world that is becoming increasingly unfamiliar. One woman once said of her husband, "He would climb inside of me if he could."

Shadowing has much in common with sundowning and wandering; it is a deep response, not conscious, but instinctive. The place in all of us that needs safety, love, and comfort produces this struggle. The middle stages of progressive dementias are deeply emotional; there is no way to truly calm those who need this reassurance. Anger, fear, and grief get fused with love and the instinct to live. The end result is stepping out of the shower face to face with someone you love, yet who exhausts you. In our home, often an elder will seek out one caregiver when it is a tough day and spend hours just inches away from that person. But we get to go home at the end of the day.

Assisted living caregivers are able to switch off and disappear when the need for space arises. A lone caregiver at home can't do this. While pets, visitors, and certain tasks can buy a caregiver a few moments of space, they do not stop the shadowing. Medication does at times lower the volume if someone is angry, anxious, or emotional. But medication does not make the need disappear. Some people get beyond this as they get deeper into the disease, but others do not. There is only one solution: respite for the caregiver.

Time away to have one's own life and space is a necessity. Sometimes an elder will be angry at the disease, and the shadowed caregiver becomes the place for all this anger to go. This is not safe. Exhaustion, illness, and an inability to judge safety hit caregivers hard in these situations. Day programs, where the elder has peers and the caregiver is not the center of the universe, can help. But if a caregiver still has someone they love following them around yelling, crying, or being fearful for several hours a day, placement can become the only option. Again, this is not failure on the caregiver's part; this is the disease.

In certain people, the need to be near someone fuses with an inability to process the stimulation of being near people, and no amount of calming music, soft words, or peaceful environment can give that elder peace. The wiring in the brain does not allow for that person to be calmed. Sometimes, this can be a health issue, a response to infection. But if there is none, caregivers must be honest about how they are holding up. I wish with all my heart that there were an approach or medicine or system that could make this easy. There is not.

The husband of a woman whom we cared for once said, "She does this the hard way." Despite the fact that the woman had amazing caregivers, a loving husband, a beautiful home, a smart doctor, and medications, all they could offer were a small amount of comfort and rare moments of freedom from dementia. No amount of love, care, or kindness was able to make her process an easy road. What she ended up with was many good people who just stayed by her. Now and then, that is as good as it gets.

Deep Alzheimer's

Alzheimer's disease is a full-body process. Our brain directs the ebb and flow of everything our body must do to be alive. When that ability to direct begins to fade, many changes take place. Elders will face an increasing need for physical assistance. Incontinence, poor balance, difficulty eating, risk of falling, and hygiene problems all require direct, hands-on care, which can spark resistance or confusion in the elder. When training staff, we frequently have them feed each other or attempt to put a shirt on each other. Caregivers need to appreciate just how invasive it can feel to have someone help with very personal care. Resistance, frustration, and misinterpretation are not "behaviors"; they are normal responses to a difficult situation. This applies to caregivers, too.

I would advise health care professionals, especially doctors, counselors, social workers, and nurses, to show balance and compassion with families around this. I can recall several instances when spouses or adult children were brought to tears when faced with one of two extremes—one is to instantly jump to medicate an elder, and the other is to instantly assume that the family must have a "problem with their approach."

Medication can at times be an act of kindness. Sometimes it allows elders to simply be comfortable inside their own skin. However, the medication discussion needs to come with a clear and direct dialogue about side effects and the fact that the drug may or may not work. Realism is kindness.

The other extreme, the assumption that caregivers are doing something wrong when they encounter difficulties in attempting to provide hands-on care, only increases the guilt, fatigue, and frustration that so many already feel. If a caregiver is bringing up problems with personal care in a doctor's or therapist's office, chances are really good that they have already tried many approaches—begged and pleaded, tried different times of day, offered snacks, etc. Despite their best efforts, these caregivers can get into problems that could easily become unsafe or unhealthy. Some elders in their fight with dementia are unable to tolerate even the most graceful and compassionate personal care. Jesus, Buddha, or Mother Teresa would have a hard time helping some of them shower or change their underwear. I don't mean to challenge anyone's faith here, but to make the point that caregivers have to show love and patience with themselves as well. Again, realism is kindness.

Some of the same approaches of soft distractions used with sundowning can also help in personal care. I recommend making the environment simple and calming, and trying not to rush, unless the elder just wants to get done and out. I have seen caregivers take a handful of candy into the shower with people: one candy, wash the feet; one candy, wash the arms; one candy, wash the back—you get the picture. Modesty can be an issue, but a person can actually get quite clean with a towel over the lap or chest.

Caregivers must be realistic about what they can do. Care for incontinence and bathing is hard physical work. Altering the physical environment with handicap grab bars and non-slip mats can be helpful, but the caution here is similar to that of making alterations to prevent wandering—caregivers must be comfortable living with them as well. Caregivers are always part of the equation. (In addition, consulting a physical therapist or home health provider about placement of bars, etc., is a good idea.)

Many caregivers work with people who outweigh them or are taller than them. This can be unsafe. Caregivers must know their own limits and have emergency backup plans. It is highly stressful for an elder when a caregiver is injured or sick. But even if the person needing care is the same size or smaller, the body mechanics can be tough. The risk for falling is high, especially if an elder is resistant, and incontinence care can be relentless. Consulting a physical therapist can be helpful. The Alzheimer's Association also offers classes that can be a great help to caregivers.

Another feature of both hygiene and incontinence care goes back to the discussion about stimulation. Many people with dementia become very, very sensitive. The old fairy tale of the princess and the pea comes to mind. Water and washing up can be this way for an elder with dementia—nothing feels quite right. But complaints of too hot, too cold, or too rough often mean it's all just too much to process. This can feel like a recurring Goldilocks scenario, with the caregiver struggling to get it "just right." The way I try to empathize is to remember the feeling of a migraine headache, or a hangover: The light is too bright, the noise is too loud, the environment is disorienting, and everything and everyone is irritating. Being cranky is not personal—it just is.

Twilight

Hygiene care, incontinence, and shadowing are all part of the "some things just suck" part of Alzheimer's and other dementias. The next stages entail the body and the brain losing the ability to communicate. I think of it as a difficult divorce: The brain and the body no longer talk. These changes reflect the fact that the brain is experiencing organ failure. This time is often a prolonged twilight; it is the beginning of the dying process. The brain has changed to the point that it simply no longer directs the body, and the elder drifts away from that body.

The changes are not immediate. I have seen people live for years with the inability to walk, frequent falls, problems with swallowing, fatigue, decreased eating and drinking, weight loss, recurrent infections, and stiffness. Despite how all this sounds, I also see people in this stage live graciously, surrounded by comfort and affection. The person, the soul, lives. And sometimes the expression of that soul becomes stronger during this time.

I keep a picture on my computer of two elders who live at Vista. One woman sits in a rocking chair, holding the hand of another woman with both hands, staring down at their hands. The other woman stands above her, stroking her hair. Both are very far along in their dementia. The lady in the chair no longer walks; her body is stiff. The lady who is standing can walk on some days, but on others can only sleep. Both struggle with food—one has problems swallowing, and the other seldom eats.

The woman in the chair had been anxious, starting to call out in random shrieking sounds until the other woman came and took her hand. As caregivers, our first impulse was, Should we move her? Should we protect? Instead, we allowed. The woman in the chair grew quiet for a few minutes, softly rocking; the other woman stroked her hair and spoke to her. Though their ability to speak in words had disappeared long ago, they communicated in soft sounds and laughter. The two women were the comforter and the comforted. Within a few minutes, as the woman in the chair drifted to sleep, the woman standing turned to giggle at the chickens outside the window. During those few minutes, the women shared kindness. They shared soul.

We have had a schoolteacher living with us now for seven years. When I first met this amazing woman, she was angry. She was facing a disease that was stripping away everything she had ever loved. Her amazing mind, her patience, the ability to be the family matriarch, and her ability to live with the only man she had ever loved—all were being assaulted by the enemy that was inside her. For years she fought, raged, and cried against an enemy she could never beat.

But somewhere in the midst of this war, she made a dear friend, she began to laugh again, and she found her love for children again. Peace slowly crept up on her. As she lost touch with more and more of her mind and body, she rediscovered the man she had loved for so long. She could take his hand without tears or rage; she could love again. She knows this man. He is part of her soul. She can't walk—she can barely stand. She can't remember her children or her grandchildren. She can't feed herself. But she can love. The words she speaks most often now are "Thank you" and "I love you." She says these words every time she is spoken to, every time someone takes her hand, every time she is touched. These words remind me of a prayer, an unceasing prayer to life, a victory over the enemy inside that has taken so much. Her fierce anger has given way to gratitude and love.

Love rules. Love wins.

Many Rooms in
the House of Dementia

The fact that an elder is "still in there" beneath the losses and struggles is common to all progressive dementias. Despite all that is taken away, love, creativity, wisdom, humor, and kindness remain. Many of the struggles that elders face are similar in all dementias—changes in memory, physical deterioration, emotional stress, and a body and brain that will fail. (The medications are similar as well, but this will be discussed later.) But there are differences in the various disease processes that make up progressive dementia.

Dementia branches

The *Diagnostic and Statistical Manual of Mental Disorders (DSM-5)* arranges the progressive dementias into groups, subgroups, and variations on disease process. The *DSM-5* names the following diseases as the branches of progressive dementia: Alzheimer's disease, frontotemporal neurocognitive disorder (also called Pick's Disease or frontotemporal dementia), Lewy body neurocognitive disorder, vascular dementia, dementia due to traumatic brain injury, substance/medication induced neurocognitive disorder, HIV-related neurocognitive disorder, prion diseases, Huntington's disease, unspecified dementia, and mixed dementia. Mild cognitive impairment (MCI) is also listed as a potential predecessor to Alzheimer's disease, Lewy body, and frontotemporal dementia.

Each of the processes listed above can be further broken down into types. MCI does seem to appear in depression and PTSD, and studies suggest that the chemical changes, hormonal changes, and inflammation in the brain that accompany these issues can shift MCI toward progressive dementia. MCI does not always develop into a progressive dementia; it simply presents an increased risk.

Other dementias

In his aforementioned book, Robert Levine provides a solid description of the more common disease processes that make up the progressive dementias as well as a thorough discussion on medication and treatment options. He also presents cautiously optimistic plans for reducing the risk of facing dementia in the future.

I will focus here on the processes of which I have working knowledge: mixed dementia; vascular dementia; Lewy body dementias; fronto-temporal lobe dementias, such as Pick's Disease and semantic frontal lobe dementia; and the alcohol-related EtOH dementia (literally "ethyl alcohol" or ethanol).

Mixed dementia refers to a condition that is layered with two or more disease processes, and the elder faces both. The most common combination is a vascular dementia with another disease process such as Alzheimer's. I have also worked with elders who faced an EtOH dementia in combination with an age-related dementia such as Lewy body disease or a frontal lobe dementia. In these complex situations, elders, caregivers, and medical professionals can all become frustrated. Patience and time end up being the answer. Communication is critical. Healing in progressive dementia is not a specific outcome or formula—it is comfort.

Vascular dementia

Vascular dementia is the most common dementia after Alzheimer's disease and is frequently part of mixed dementia—

50 percent of all cases have a vascular component. Vascular dementia can also be a primary diagnosis.

Approximately 20 percent of people with progressive dementia have cerebrovascular disease. Silent strokes, also called "infarcts," create bleeding within the brain, which is frequently microscopic. A TIA, or transient ischemic attack, is a term used to describe the micro-strokes in which tiny vessels break and cause bleeding within the brain, which decreases oxygen and restricts blood flow. Over time, the damage builds to the point of decreasing a person's ability to function.

Vascular dementia can cause aphasia (loss of speech), emotional issues such as anger and depression, and disturbance of both fine and gross motor skills. Many elders develop balance issues and experience increased difficulty with walking. As the disease progresses, the emotional part of the struggle can cause frustration for both elder and caregiver. Elders can seem to be stuck in a level of functioning that is hard for them to process and accept, contributing to a short fuse around personal care and the universe in general. Caregivers must remind themselves that this is a disease symptom and is not personal. The devoted daughter-in-law of one of our elders put it this way: "Mom isn't mad at any of us—she's just mad at her brain."

In our Vista ecosystem, we have had some positive results incorporating animals into the lives of elders who seem either stuck and angry or frustrated at losing verbal skills. The companionship of a creature that loves without question and does not need to talk can be invaluable. Eden Alternative has done some excellent research on the benefits of animal companions for elders. (Just being quietly present with someone who is angry can also be helpful.)

Promising research from UC Irvine suggests that vascular dementia can be stabilized in certain cases with medication and lifestyle changes. Like much of the cautious optimism in Robert Levine's book, the MEND Protocol, a complex mix of therapies, nutrition, medication, and exercise, is more effective early in the process. Moreover, compliance becomes problematic in the later stages of dementia.

The University of New Mexico, with a National Institutes of Health grant, is conducting studies on the effects of blood flow within the brain in search of ways to treat vascular dementia and Alzheimer's. The research center also has a treatment branch.

On a day-to-day basis, treatment is generally focused on preventing strokes (often with blood thinners), maintaining mental functioning, and comforting those elders dealing with depression and anger. If an elder has difficulty with walking and balance, the situation becomes more problematic. Poor or no safety awareness is an innate part of all progressive dementia, stemming from impaired executive functioning and impaired judgment. Someone with poor balance and problems with walking will simply not remember to ask for help; they may also not want help. This creates falls, and falls in combination with bleeding risk are especially dangerous. The end result is a risky and complex balancing act.

Caregivers often feel torn between the desire to slow the progression of the dementia and the risk that medication may pose. There is no clear answer to this. Finding a balance between managing the potential risk of a stroke that would worsen the dementia and the risk of a fall that could turn into a major bleeding episode is complicated. Building a healthy relationship with one's doctor who can help consider the risks and benefits is important.

The Elder Consult website offers some insights around the use of blood thinning medications in vascular dementia in a straightforward way. The Eden Alternative principles also help here: Which is going to allow for more comfort and security in day-to-day life? Atul Gawande's beautiful book *Being Mortal* explores complex medical decisions and palliative care. I have found it helpful.

While reading and asking questions is always positive, both family and professional caregivers need to trust their hearts and their own common sense. Love will lead to the best answer, and that answer may change with time.

Lewy body dementias

To say that Lewy body disease is complicated is an under-statement. The disease processes lumped under this label are complex and unpredictable. Dr. Levine begins his chapter on LBD with a quote from the *Tao Te Ching*: "Plan for the difficult while it is easy."

Getting a diagnosis as early as possible, even if it is changed later, will help both the person facing the disease and the care-givers. If a caregiver understands that medication may have the exact opposite effect that it should, they may feel a little less frustration. If a caregiver has time to create a plan for dis-rupted sleep early in the disease process, this can reduces stress and fatigue later. Connecting with a receptive doctor and get-ting a good referral to a psychiatrist or neurologist early on helps too. In many communities, waiting three or four months for an appointment with such a specialist is not unusual. One should get the referral and make the appointment even if it does not seem to be needed at the moment.

Lewy body dementia is named for protein deposits that are found deep within the gray matter of the brain. Dr. Frederich Henrich Lewy discovered this phenomenon in 1912. Until the mid-1980s, LBD was considered a rare disorder. Since then, research and brain imaging have improved, and these demen-tias are now believed to be much more common.

Lewy body dementia is an umbrella term that covers Parkin-son's dementia, Lewy body disease, and Alzheimer's disease with Lewy body variant, all of which have differences in symp-toms, progression, and response to medication. The disease process frequently includes unpredictable behavior, and there is a wide range of both physical and cognitive issues, which contributes to its complexity. The disease often strikes people in their fifties or sixties, and the progression can be more rapid than Alzheimer's disease or vascular dementia. Both the intensity of care and the cost of care are more extreme for the majority of people facing LBD.

• Problems you may face

The most common problems that elders and caregivers face with LBD are similar to those of Alzheimer's, though with a few important additions. Cognition and emotional states can fluctuate rapidly throughout the day. Many people will experience night terrors (sometimes while awake) and highly erratic sleep patterns. In his truly amazing book *The Lewy Body Soldier*, Norman McNamara shares his personal experience with LBD, writing in a direct and powerful way about his life with night terrors, hallucinations, and how it feels to be completely "there" and then "gone." He writes as a warrior, with a certain toughness about his life and this painful process.

Hallucinations can range from benign to frightening. While several people I have worked with have been able to tell me what they see, others have not. I remember a lady discussing how beautiful the deep-blue horses were in the backyard. I also remember a man trying to push the demons away. For both of these people, what they saw was absolutely real, far more real than the caregiver sitting next to them.

Fluctuations in cognition and emotion can bring on sudden aggressive behavior, which is both similar and different to the frustration, sundowning, and catastrophic reactions (exaggerated responses to stimulus) that occur in other dementia processes. Like the above, this is a deep, instinctual response; the difference is that there is an innate randomness to it. Sometimes the kind, gentle, calming responses from a caregiver just will not work. The stimulation the person is responding to may not be one the caregiver can change. It is not a specific thing in the environment or approach that triggers the response; it just is. The situation can end quickly or become pro-longed. Because the stimulation that a person is responding to may be internal, shifting someone's attention is much more dif-ficult. Norman McNamara describes one incident: He could hear his wife's soft, reassuring voice, but it seemed very far away. She was holding his hand, but he could not reach her to calm down.

Caregivers should not blame themselves for being unable to calm or distract someone in the midst of a behavioral episode. While a calming approach can help, the disease process has its own life. Working with a sensitive doctor who will listen can help. However, LBD is difficult to medicate as there is a tendency for drugs to produce a "paradoxical reac-tion." In a home with a lone caregiver, where a medication meant to calm aggressive behavior does the opposite, the re-sults can be really bad.

Some people with LBD will develop the physical problems associated with Parkinson's disease: tremors, stiffness, or weak-ness, in addition to heart-related symptoms such as lowered blood pressure, edema in the legs and feet, and some light-headedness. Some elders face more of the physical issues, some more behavioral, and still others a combination of both. Many elders do not get diagnosed until they are deep into the de-mentia process and are having obvious hallucinations or phys-ical problems.

• Depression

Depression, which Norman McNamara calls "the concrete overcoat," is frequently part of this process. "Concrete over-coat" is a haunting image. The weight and immobilizing quality of depression is a struggle for anyone, but adding LBD to it makes good medical care crucial for comfort and safety. How-ever, alternative therapies such as music, art, poetry, and exer-cise can build self-esteem, release emotions, and allow elders to shift their focus to a positive direction. Connecting to other people through support groups, dementia cafes, assisted living settings, and faith communities can be helpful in offsetting depression. These therapies and social connections apply to caregivers as well; they also need to tend to their emotions.

• Accepting change

For caregivers, this means they cannot face this alone. It also means an elder's needs may change as the disease progresses. This applies to families as well as to facility staff. Over the years, we at Vista Living Care have cared very well for elders facing LBD; we have also had to refer some to more clinical programs as the disease progressed. The work that our awesome nurses and caregivers do so beautifully is to provide a home that is loving, social, natural, and connected to life. For most elders, this balance is perfect. However, we are not a skilled nursing facility. Sometimes people with LBD progress in ways that require highly structured medical care and access to a physician on a twenty-four hour basis. This is not predictable; elders may live comfortably for years in a setting like ours, or the disease may change their needs within a few months. Each elder is different.

This can happen for many reasons. Issues such as increased difficulty managing Parkinson's symptoms, behavioral issues that create a danger to oneself or others, and more extreme reactions to stimulation can cause an elder to need medical intervention on a continual basis. Stimulation is even more complex in LBD because of the hallucinations. This disease process can decrease an elder's tolerance for noise, touch, and activity, resulting in someone who feels constantly overstimulated and on edge. Often these elders desperately want to be comforted but cannot tolerate being close to others. Medical interventions and a highly structured routine can provide comfort; peaceful environments can also help.

We worked with one gentleman who found refuge in a residential hospice program, which at first seemed like an odd choice. Most elders who were as strong as he was at the time would have been restless and a bored in that setting, but its low level of stimulation was comforting for him. We need to be open to the fact that someone may need to change placements at different stages in their disease process. This does not mean that anyone failed; it is just the disease. Psychiatrist Carl Hammerschlag once said, "Healing is what works." This is true for all people with dementia. Healing is what brings comfort, safety, and connection. This may change over time, and it may be unexpected or unusual.

• Signals for end-of-life care

One of the amazing doctors we work with, Toni Camp, M.D., has explained that some people with LBD will experience a rapid increase in unpredictable, aggressive behaviors prior to a severe physical decline. This can result in an end-of-life situation. Caregivers should keep their eyes open for physical changes that may accompany or precede the behavioral change. Decreased appetite, recurring infections, and loss of the ability to walk alone are some common things to watch for. What we tell families is to be aware of changes that seem to come in clusters. If several parts of someone's life change at the same time, it is likely another step in the process of the disease. With all dementias, it is important to have previously discussed, as a family, what kinds of care and what level of care is wanted at the end of life.

Frontal lobe dementias

Frontal lobe dementias are a cluster of related disease processes that greatly change the brain and the life of the elder that brain belongs to. As with LBD, what is called frontal lobe dementia, Pick's disease, or frontotemporal lobe disease is often a cluster of disease processes that actually affect the brain differently while manifesting some common physical, cognitive, and behavioral changes. These processes are also complex.

First discovered in 1892 by Dr. Arnold Pick, frontotemporal dementia, or FTD, is still the subject of intense research. A recent study by researchers at UC San Francisco has identified distinct variations in brain atrophy in patients diagnosed with FTD. This information might not help the everyday person facing this disease, but it does begin the process of finding a way to intervene and respond to the cascade of brain death. It also explains its wide array of symptoms.

In simple terms, what happens in all processes under the FTD umbrella is that parts of the brain basically wither away. This usually begins in the frontal and temporal lobes. While this is common to all progressive dementias, the speed and severity separates these processes from others. The age of onset also differs. The majority of people diagnosed with FTD (60 percent) are younger than sixty-five; the average age at diagnosis is forty-seven.

FTD affects someone's life in many ways. Howard Kirschner, M.D., writes that often the first sign may not be memory loss, but a change in the ability to connect with the outside world. This shows up in many ways: loss of inhibition, social withdrawal, disregard for hygiene, delusions of a suspicious or paranoid nature, increase in alcohol or prescription drugs, overeating, the eating of nonfood items, changes in sexual behavior, hypersexuality, decrease in language skills, increased difficulty with walking, becoming "accident prone," spatial disorientation or getting lost, changes in eye movement, bad judgment, muscle stiffness and soreness, and memory loss.

• Depression and addiction

There are two common and confusing warning signs of FTD: depression and addiction. Many of the early signs of this process can seem like depression. Addiction, weight gain, suspicion, social withdrawal, and changes in hygiene are all linked to depression. If someone has faced a trauma such as the death of a loved one, a divorce, a job loss, a major move, or another event that can create deep grief, they should get support. If counseling and antidepressant medication is not helpful, they need a medical work-up and a visit to a neurologist.

Something frequently seen in emergency rooms is the effects of a person self-medicating the beginning of progressive dementia with alcohol and prescription anxiety or pain medications. Velma and I have both pulled elders out of emergency rooms who are in very bad shape with this combination. FTD is usually the dementia that does this. With FTD, judgment is often changed before memory—someone feels like they should function, but they can't. The natural response is to do whatever it takes to feel better. The problem is that often "whatever it takes" ends up making the problem much, much worse. If someone who has never abused drugs or alcohol begins to abuse, FTD could be the cause. (Extreme overeating might also occur.) The end result is a circle where each problem feeds the other and increases the damage to the brain and body.

• Structure and freedom

Here is another feature we have seen with FTD: Someone goes into a home like Vista Living Care and does really well. With the structure and support to be healthy, clean, and creative, they eat right, they get sober. They get better. The person who was previously in the ER in a fetal position, or being pulled from their home by Adult Protective Services, becomes a leader in the assisted living. But memory is not the biggest problem in their life. They feel like the caregivers are telling them what to do. Soon the person convinces their family, friends, and doctor that they can function with more independence. So they move to an apartment or go home—only to crash and burn within a few weeks. The bottom drops out of their life.

Often, people with any kind of dementia function well because of the structure and people around them. Twenty-four-hour care allows them to have independence and freedom, rather than the in-and-out care they might receive at home, if at all. Take away the help, and the disease runs their life. As I see it, if it's not broken, don't fix it. If someone is doing really well with help, they probably need that help. This is where the "not like those people" can cause a lot of pain for everyone. Anyone who loves someone with dementia or any other terminal illness wants a miracle. We all want it to be better. We all want it to go away. But it doesn't. What we get are times of peace and joy that may last longer than we expect. We should love these times, not mess with them.

• Beauty and the brain

Another strange and honestly beautiful quirk of FTD is creativity. I know this disease is hard, but inside all people is something resilient and life affirming, even in the face of dementia. Later in this book I write about a lady who began to draw as she lost her ability to use words. FTD has a variant called "semantic frontal lobe dementia." This is the enemy she faces through the beauty of her art. Yes, the enemy will win. In the meantime, she can have small victories on paper with color and line.

Becoming more creative while living with FTD is not unusual. Researchers at UC San Francisco have done extensive studies of people with FTD variants and found art to be one of the most effective therapies. Creating art allows people to focus on something other than their tangled emotions. It allows them to express what there may not be words for. It is a strange gift that many people who were never creative in their "functional" lives become creative in the midst of dementia. I see this as a way of holding on to life and hope. Lines and color on paper can become times of peace and joy.

Music is also helpful if an elder can handle the stimulation of sound without becoming overloaded. At Vista Living, we use music as a behavior intervention, changing it several times a day according to the mood of the house. For the majority of elders who face dementia, music is possibly the best way to reach them as long as we are sensitive to their needs.

• Being open to changes

Just as Lewy body dementia can at times progress in ways that need more clinical care, FTD can as well. Certain aspects such as hypersexuality, pica (the eating of nonfood items), muscle stiffness, pain, or falls can become safety issues for both the person with FTD and those around them. However, many people with FTD do not have severe behavioral or safety issues. One must simply be aware. Adapting a family home to caring for people with these issues is often unrealistic.

Highly structured—even secure—environments with round-the-clock nurses and doctors in the building are not always restrictive, as someone without dementia may perceive. Sometimes the structure is freeing for the person with FTD, allowing them to be grounded in ways that they simply could not be in a looser setting. FTD tends to progress in drops and plateaus. An elder may seem stable, functioning at a certain level for months, and then go into what feels like a freefall, only to plateau again. This is hard. There is grieving at each drop, and anxiety at each plateau. Caregivers need support at these times.

Addiction-related dementia

Dementia related to addictions, often called EtOH, is similar to other progressive dementias in how it affects a person's life.

Short-term memory loss, emotional stress and fluctuations, and general confusion are common. Long-term addiction, like long-term depression, PTSD, or other mental illness, tends to open the door for dementia. Some elders do not show cognitive problems until years after they have stopped the addictive behavior. This and many other parts of progressive dementia are deeply unfair.

The elders I have worked with who face this usually have mixed dementia. The substance abuse history basically complicates another age-related dementia. A complication that can be connected to this is a person craving alcohol or drugs years after quitting. Memory is going backward; the person with dementia may be returning to a time in their lives when they were using. Families, doctors, and assisted living staff end up becoming gatekeepers in these situations. For the majority of elders, this phase, like anxiety or anger, does pass as the disease progresses.

Complex compassion

Dementia of any kind is a hard process. When I was in graduate school, we were taught to help, look for solutions, and empower people to make things better. But in the work I have done for the past twenty years, there are no solutions. Sometimes empowerment is helping an elder or family member learn how to let go. Sometimes it means fighting even when you know that losing is the only end. Making progress means something entirely different in the face of progressive dementia than it does when one is studying to be a therapist. Progress in dementia is comfort, moments of connection, creativity, joy, and love. It is also facing the ugly, uncontrolled, unrelenting disease. It is everything in the process, including helplessness.

While the research I have done for this book gives me hope, it still leaves millions of people who are in the process now just trying to put the pieces together. And that process is becoming more complex. There are increasingly more openness, more honesty, and better science, along with the challenge of caring for people with dignity and love. There is the shock at what kind of resources that will take. In the end, there are also people who show amazing courage and compassion every day. There is love.

Food Is Not Always Love

Food, glorious food. . .
Live to eat. Eat to live.

Food blogs, food posts, Food Network, cookbooks, celebrity chefs, Chopped.

Farm to table, fast food nation, slow food revolution, food deserts, food justice.

Paleo diet, South Beach diet, gourmet food trucks, food tourism.

It is safe to say that Americans are more than a little obsessed with food. We tend to put many emotions into how food is grown, purchased, prepared, presented, offered, and shared. Guilt, love, fear, and stress may all be expressed through food. Food can be fun, and it can also be a struggle. Food can be healing, both physically and emotionally, and it can also create problems and cause discomfort. Food can be a connection to others. People can also become disconnected to food.

Dementia adds more complexity to food for many reasons. During the disease process, the brain changes, neurons die, messages get crossed, and the body begins to relate to food in different ways. Elders who struggle with Alzheimer's will often lose weight, even when they are eating well. The early stages of frontal lobe dementia can cause behavioral changes that create obesity and open the door to becoming diabetic. Medications can cause nausea, decrease appetite, and change the taste of food. An elder may develop food cravings that do not make sense with their life history. An elder may desire the food they ate in childhood. An elder can relive an eating disorder from their teens. Like all other relationships in life, dementia changes our relationship with food.

Food is food, love is love

I am not a nutritionist, a dietician, or a chef. My perspective is that of a caregiver, a sister, and a friend. There are some wonderful studies about diet, health, and aging out there—this chapter is not that. Rather, it is about the day-in and day-out relationship with eating and food that I see in my work with elders and with my brother as he faces a terminal illness. What I have are everyday stories of what eating can mean in the face of a changing body and brain.

Nutrition and dementia are an odd combination. At some point, every calorie is a good one. At another point, a person's body will simply not want or need as much food. For families, food can feel like a way to help, like something we can control. The truth is that this is an illusion. We often can't control the relationship that the person we are caring for has with food. We can support, offer alternatives, and be there, but ultimately we cannot control it. The question then becomes, How do we as caregivers do our best in the face of so many factors we cannot control? The answer is, We listen to the person we are caring for.

Listening to someone with dementia or someone who is terminally ill is about much more than words. We have to pay attention and be present with that person in respect and kindness even when they are not doing what makes us feel better. This is a language that is more than words; part of knowing how to deal with eating is learning that language. Is someone smiling when they eat certain foods? Are they clenching their teeth or pushing you away when you try to help them eat? Do they seem lost when holding a fork or spoon? Do they grimace or choke when eating? Do they seem distracted by whatever noises, light, or movement are around them during a meal?

Does food calm them or cause them distress? Are we making food decisions for the person we are caring for, or for ourselves?

Fries and happiness

Velma and I worked with a caring, bright director several years ago who was very concerned about healthy eating. She shared concerns about fats, cholesterol, and the fact that our menu included some fried foods. (This was before paleo diets and good fats were the fad.) These were great observations that came from a loving heart. The catch was that she was working with a group of elders who were in the later stages of dementia and were prone to losing weight. This group, like many other people, really loved their fries. They also loved their cake and ice cream, but that is another story. It took many discussions to come to the conclusion that although we served salads, the fries would not go away.

There is a class of food I call "happiness and joy food." This means something different for every person, but for someone who is losing the fight with a major illness, this is the food that matters. The nutritional value becomes secondary to the emotional comfort and pleasure of the food on the plate.

Dementia stages and eating

Food is a part of life where the stages of dementia do matter. The Alzheimer's Association recommends following a Mediterranean diet for all of us who are trying to keep our brains healthy, including people in the early stages of dementia. National Geographic, the World Health Organization, and the National Institutes of Health have all done excellent research on the "Blue Zones" of the world where cultures enjoy both long life expectancy and good health. These studies show the benefits of combining good food, exercise, love, purpose, and faith for long, healthy lives. (Dementia still exists in these places; the odds against it are just better.) I recently came across a wonderful book by Francie Healy on cooking for a healthy brain, *Eat to Beat Alzheimer's*, which has some great information and excellent recipes.

But all of this research is more relevant for the general population than for many of the elders I care for. Somewhere in the middle stages of dementia, everything changes. At some point, all bets are off, and the disease directs an elder's life. Life changes here. Food changes here. Brains, bodies, and taste buds no longer communicate in logical, sensible ways. This is the time for being with someone, for accepting them as they are. The goal changes to comfort. And that comfort can come in some very strange ways.

The chiletarian and other odd changes

We cared for an elder who had been a meditation teacher and vegan for decades. He was eating poorly. His caregivers tried serving him every vegan meal they could imagine, but to no avail. One day at lunch, one of the elders sitting with him left her bowl of chile (not vegan) on the table and walked away. (I am talking New Mexico *chile* here, not to be confused with chili.) He took the chile, ate it all, and demanded seconds. That day, we witnessed the birth of a "chiletarian." Red chile or green chile, with beef, pork, or beans, in Frito pies or enchiladas, he would eat anything with chile. Another elder loved all her food with honey or pancake syrup. In fact, many elders consider dessert to be the primary food group; beyond concern for diabetics, the pleasure of food is all important.

We have found that flexibility is essential. Most elders can focus on meals earlier in the day, which makes breakfast and lunch the most substantial meals at Vista. Certain elders become grazers, meaning they eat small amounts throughout the day and night instead of full meals. Engaging an elder in the process of cooking can also increase eating.

For two decades, Vista Living Care has specialized in the care of those living with Alzheimer's and dementia. Our philosophies are intentional and build around the needs of our elders. Our kitchens and meal-time philosophies are an example of this and are far from the cafeteria settings where food is cooked behind doors and often carted through hallways before being served.

At Vista, we cook our food from scratch with an open kitchen. Being able to smell, see, and interact with food prior to eating helps elders engage with food and acts as a cue to eat. Smell is the sense that stays intact the longest in the brain and is the most deeply connected to memory, awareness, and cognition. Think of how comforting the smell of chicken soup is on a winter day, or how nice it is to watch someone cook, chatting with them as they wash vegetables or season a sauce. These are universal human feelings that help people eat.

Taste buds tend to drift back to infancy as the disease progresses. Velma uses the phrase "soft, smooth, sweet." This is a good description for ice cream, yogurt, smoothies, puddings, flan, chilled fruit, and other comforting foods that are easy on the stomach. Often they move from being desserts to sides to main dishes as elders reach the late stages of progressive dementia.

Ensure, Boost, and other supplements

It is common to use supplements such as Ensure and Boost as eating decreases. These come in puddings, shakes, and clear drinks. They are helpful in that they can create comfort, and the clear drinks help with dehydration. These nutrition supplements help keep skin healthy and may increase the ability to heal if there is a wound or a sore. They also can be a way for someone to maintain energy a bit longer. These supplements can also be used as a replacement for vitamin and mineral pills if an elder refuses to take them. While the drinks may not be an exact match, it is a step in the right direction. Some people enjoy these drinks, others not so much. Naturally, the person we are caring for gets to decide—if they do not want to take them, they should never be forced.

Medical interventions

Two questions come up around eating or lack of eating. One is whether to use medications or medical marijuana to increase appetite, and the other is whether to use feeding tubes. Both are questions for a doctor and are important to discuss with an elder's family. States have different laws regarding medical marijuana, and although research is being done on its use in dementia care, it is mostly in other countries. Whatever allows for more comfort is what is helpful and healing.

We worked with a lady who, in the middle stages of Alzheimer's, began to act out an eating disorder. We found ourselves caring for a seventy-something-year-old bulimic. Her doctor, who had hospice and cancer experience, prescribed Marinol, an artificial THC used in cancer care. It helped. The lady was able to eat in a normal, relaxed way. She gained a little weight and returned to her happy, charming self. After several months, her dementia took her beyond any of the ghosts she had in her past around food, and she no longer needed the medication. This does not mean this approach would work for everyone. Medication, like food, can become complex and unpredictable for someone with middle to advanced dementia. It is important to work closely with a doctor on any medication issues.

I have not worked with feeding tubes. In our state, to have a feeding tube, a person must reside at home or in a skilled nursing facility, not in assisted living such as Vista Living Care. I have great respect for both hospice and palliative care—this kind of care has made my brother's life better. But I also respect people who feel the preservation of life is always needed. We all find our way through this with love. There are many choices. I just stress the need for caregivers to be very clear about why they are making the choices they make.

Palliative approach

One of our dear friends and colleagues, Denys Cope, wrote the book *Dying: A Natural Passage*. In this sensitive book, she compares the stages of death to pregnancy and giving birth. Her background as a hospice nurse allows her to discuss the decrease in eating in a practical yet gentle way. She describes how the appetite decreases as the body loses the energy to process food. The lowered intake is a natural way to create comfort. For many people with dementia or other health issues, this process of decreasing intake can begin far earlier than expected and last far longer.

Both my brother and a few of our elders eat little. Morgan will still have days in which he eats more than one meal, but this is usually followed by a day or so of minimal eating. He still loves going to restaurants, but that meal may be the only meal of the day, and he usually won't finish it. For almost two decades, I have sat with families and gently explained this process. Despite this, it is painful to face. Morgan's nurse gently explained this process to me, and something he said has stayed with me: We should follow his lead and not push or assume that he is feeling what we would be feeling.

Morgan has been comfortable and happy in his life of minimal eating since April 2017. He has lost weight but is still strong enough to enjoy his pets, movies, friends, and music. I still struggle with the desire to control his choices, with the guilt of not being able to fix everything, and with the fear of losing him. I still wonder if I'm doing enough. But he is okay. And so are our elders who eat little.

Caregivers and food

One of the ironies of the universe is that while many caregivers work with elders who are in the phase of life when food is about pleasure and comfort, we ourselves are of an age when we need to be careful about what we eat. This is tough when we are caring for someone for whom every calorie is a good one. Stress-eating more as the person we care for eats less creates its own problems. Likewise, if your elder is not eating, don't join them. Understanding that we need different things from the person we care for is important in many, many ways. Food is just one of them.

Caregivers often neglect to take the time to eat properly and forget that their health is critical to the person they are caring for. Yes, every book, social worker, support group, counselor, and well-meaning friend out there preaches self-care, often to the point of making caregivers want to strangle them. But there is a reason for this: None of us can give what we haven't got. We also are not helping by trying to will the people we care for into being someone they no longer are. We are not helping when we beat ourselves up for not being able to cure a disease process that more than a century of medical science has not beaten. We as caregivers do not control; we love, we work, and most importantly, we are there.

Another Kind of Love Story—
Sexuality and Dementia

Just another love story

He was tall and tanned, with big brown eyes and thick white hair. He loved music, dancing, and animals of all kinds. Every morning he read *The New York Times,* and every evening he watched over his chickens, peacocks, and goats. He was a businessman turned gentleman farmer. He loved to talk and was always in charge. He was in his nineties.

She was tall, slim, and blonde, with perfect cheekbones. She talked and laughed constantly. She loved people, music, clothes, dancing, and life. She believed in love. She was in her seventies.

A friend takes credit for introducing them. He says with pride, "I introduced my ex-wife to her new husband. They are perfect." He was right. They lit up the world around them.

They both got to forget forgetting and remember dancing. Deep connection became their lives. They brought gossip, joy, and laughter to the house. He was able to spend the last few months of his life deeply in love with this beautiful lady, and she gets to remember him: "He was a good man…kind…my man." The lady's eyes fill with tears, but she also smiles. She remembers loving and being loved.

The couple in this story, which was written up in *Natural Awakenings Magazine* in 2013, met and fell in love at Vista. They were both deep into their fight with dementia when they met, but their relationship was not part of a disease. It was a triumph over disease. It was a deeply loving human connection.

Love, sex, and dementia

All too often there is a tendency to look at an elder with dementia who feels love and sexual attraction as a misguided collection of needs instead of a human being capable of being in relationship with another. The couple in the above story had a real relationship. They loved each other. Did they need help with some basic parts of their lives? Yes. Did they always get the other one's name right? No. They ended up being "sweetheart" and "my darling" for the most part, which sounds like some other couples I know.

Love, sex, and relationship in dementia can be complicated and confusing. As someone who is divorced, I can say this stuff is complicated for everybody. Clearly, many people get confused around their relationships. According to *Statista*, Match.com Group's dating revenue was $1.28 billion in 2017. Clearly, we are willing to spend a lot of money and time to find joy in that part of their lives.

Does dementia bring special sets of problems to love and sex? Yes, dementia brings special sets of problems to everything, from eating breakfast, to tying shoes, to falling in love. Being the spouse of someone facing dementia is one of the longest, toughest, and most loving journeys that any human being can face. In her wonderful book *Dr. Ruth's Guide for the Alzheimer's Caregiver: How to Care for Your Loved One without Getting Overwhelmed. . .and without Doing It All Yourself*, Dr. Ruth Westheimer discusses sexuality in early-stage dementia for spouses. She takes an approach that I love: Be sensible, honest, direct, and sensitive. Don't let this disease take away tenderness and connection. Pat Snyder, in her book *Treasures in the Darkness: Extending the Early Stage of Lewy Body Dementia, Alzheimer's, and Parkinson's Disease*, discusses how beneficial couples counseling was for her and her husband as they faced the early stages of his battle with LBD. Both books address the importance of putting the person before the disease.

This issue is not necessarily any easier for adult children or friends. The chances of the person with dementia being confused about sex or acting in ways that might make others uncomfortable are probably pretty good. But the chances that that confusion or action is not a major problem and can easily be redirected are also pretty good. This is especially true as someone moves into the middle stages of the disease process. Many people with dementia might make off-color remarks, undress, or make passes at people, including their own adult children. Some people with dementia become more affectionate; others may become more clingy and anxious. Much of this behavior has as much to do with memory loss and changes in executive functioning as with sexuality.

Someone with dementia will not necessarily think about sex more or have a higher drive; they just lack the filter that prevents them from expressing the random thoughts that go through their head at any given moment. Elders can also become confused about who someone is and just what their relationship to that person is. So if you look like your mother or father—like the wife or husband of that elder with dementia—they might see you as that person, not as their child. Try not to be horrified or frightened. This is not bizarre behavior, and it is not hypersexuality. It is just a problem with the time, person, and context processing part of their brain. You are caught in a time warp. The response of the people around them is what is important here. Remember that honestly, this is probably not a big deal. Responding in a calm, natural, and graceful way decreases stress. Gently shifting their attention to something else is usually the best path.

Health and comfort

Other health issues can be expressed in what may seem to be sexual behavior. Undressing and excess masturbation can both be signs of beginning incontinence, urinary infections, ill-fitting clothing, or skin irritations. Comfort and good health need to be addressed first. Getting these in line allows the rest to fall into place. Because changes in any behavior can be related to physical causes, we should start there. Rule out infections—check the skin. Estrogen and progesterone cream can also be useful for women.

Both women and men will tend to undress as part of becoming incontinent. This is not a sexual behavior; it is related more to being unable to perform tasks in sequential order. It helps to approach these issues in a logical way. These issues usually have solutions, and often the solutions are simply about personal care.

Hypersexuality

During my years of working with dementia, I have worked with only a handful of elders who would be considered hypersexual in clinical terms. This is different from the elder who took the Vista Living Care owner by the hand to tell him how beautiful his eyes were, or the gentlemen who agreed to go to bed if our director would go with him. (By the time he got to his room, he had forgotten the entire conversation.) These actions fall into the category of saying whatever comes to mind in the moment.

Elders with dementia who seek out each other's company in assisted living, who hold hands, snuggle, watch (or sleep through) movies together, and kiss each other good morning at breakfast are not being hypersexual. They just like each other and are happier when they are together. Their relationship includes confusion, but it is an otherwise normal relationship. The couple may need support and redirection in addition to privacy, but it is still a positive, life affirming connection.

Hypersexual behavior is different. It is more closely related to wandering and shadowing, or aggressive and possessive behaviors. It is sexual behavior that is expressed in an uncomfortable, anxiety-ridden, highly repetitive, aggressive way. It is also not a conscious behavior. The person who is struggling with this is not a predator. There is no ill intention or meanness involved; it is an issue of the brain and body not functioning or processing. It is also manageable with good care. Working with a doctor or psychiatrist is useful. We have seen a combination of oral progesterone and antidepressant or a low dose of an antipsychotic medication prescribed in positive ways to comfort someone. It is important to communicate carefully about this with the elder's physician because of medication side effects and the changing disease process. Certain medications can have side effects that create an increase in sex drive or anxiety, so looking closely at medication history and polypharmacy issues (the concurrent use of multiple medications) is important as well.

Hypersexual behavior can occur with many types of dementia and can be an issue for both men and women. Treating this is important because this set of behaviors is not only uncomfortable for the people around the hypersexual person, but are also quite uncomfortable for the elder with the behaviors.

An elderly gentleman we worked with struggled with this issue. He would become grabby, irritable, and possessive. His peers did not want to be around him, which made the problem worse. He was lonely; he was uncomfortable in his own skin. With the cooperation of his primary physician, family, and a consulting psychiatrist, along with the attention of our awesome nurse, he was able to relax. The fact that our staff was calm, honest, and non-judgmental encouraged his healing. He went from being irritable, lonely, and aggressive to being a pleasant, funny, and sought-after lunch and dinner companion. In his life, the phrase "better living through chemistry" was true.

It really is okay

Honestly, most of the "problems" with dementia and sexuality have to do with the people who don't have dementia. We *do* need to protect elders. There *is* abuse and neglect out there.

But there is also some serious ageism, hyper-vigilance, and prudishness out there. This is a really hard process for spouses, families, and friends. One of the things I am most proud of at Vista Living Care is how well we educate families and friends; it makes us who we are. Being as honest as possible in a loving way causes many problems to simply evaporate and gives us the room to provide loving care for everyone in the process. Learning about how the person you love is changing makes many things more normal. It allows empathy to happen. Empathy does not mean trying to fix every odd thing the person you love may do. Empathy means respecting that person as a human being who may find comfort in the love of a friend who also has dementia. That can be a hard thing for a spouse or a child to see, but with honesty and support, it can also be a comforting thing.

The wife of one of our elders told us during a family conference that she actually felt joy that her husband had "found happiness" in a companion he met at Vista. She also explained that she felt less guilt for her own time with their grandchildren that her husband was unable to share, and for the fact that she loved her independence. Her husband having a friend allowed her the freedom to love her life without hesitation.

There are so many things that dementia takes away, but love in all its many forms is not one of them. It doesn't matter if someone is straight or gay, male or female, where they grew up, what language they speak, or what the makeup of their family is. Love doesn't get taken away. You get to love. Even when you are dying, and maybe especially when you are dying, you have the freedom to love. The boundaries that separate people change.

Sometimes a spouse without dementia will fall in love with someone else as their spouse fades away from them. That can be a good thing. Love is never wrong. One of the more touching things I have seen was when the husband of a woman we cared for became involved with another woman, and his new partner then became involved in the wife's care. She really wanted to help care for the last woman her partner had loved. He loved his wife who had late-stage dementia, so she was part of their life together. The new partner also loved the man's wife; she took care of both of them as best she could. Our lady did not lose a marriage—she gained a protective, engaged friend. The three of them were a family. The world may get smaller with dementia, but in the right place with the right people, love gets bigger.

The story of Jose and Nelleke

We worked with two families from very different backgrounds who became close because their parents became a couple. In a world without Alzheimer's, these two elders might have never met. He was a miner; she was a doctor. He was divorced and widowed, a lapsed Catholic with two sons and a daughter-in-law who was a guardian angel. She had raised six children, run a family medical practice, and was a devoted Methodist. They were Jose and Nelleke.

Their families both had the wisdom to respect the choice their parents made. The families would sit together at holidays. They became one big Dutch, Northern New Mexico Hispanic family for a few years. Nelleke's youngest "baby girl," a widow who had become her mother's best friend and caregiver, accepted her mother's friend as part of the family. Jose's daughter-in-law and sons were happy that he had this nice lady in his life. Despite dementia, three languages, eight kids, and two faiths, these two elders were always a positive influence on one another. They looked out for one another. He reminded her to drink more water. She scolded him when he tried to skip his medication or did not want to shave. He almost always did what she asked. She kept him awake in church. He told stories in English and Spanish that made her laugh. She was a good listener and made sure he was polite. He would call her his "old lady." She would elbow him and laugh, and whisper to him in Dutch. He had no idea what she was saying, but it always made him smile. They were always near each other. They both made each other more calm and happy.

When she passed away suddenly, he changed. Something inside him that had held off the dementia and confusion began to let go. He was never as strong after that. They are both gone now. I am grateful to be a small part of the time they had together. I will always be grateful that I had the chance to know them. I will always be proud of our home and their families for accepting these two as a real relationship. I am proud to work in a place where love rules.

Medicine, Madness, and Miracles

\Not completely science fiction

It is the year 2078. It has been forty years since the Great Care Crash, also known as the "Silver Revolution" of the 2030s. A moderately effective vaccine for Alzheimer's has been in use for ten years now, and cases have decreased by almost 15 percent. It is recommended to be given at age thirty with a booster dose every seven to ten years thereafter. Three additional medications are given to people who present signs of memory loss after forty. This has decreased the number of people who lose the ability to function, especially for dementias such as Lewy body disease and Pick's disease. There is still no cure for dementia, but researchers have worked hard to make up for the sins of the past.

The United States and many other countries have made supporting elders and caregivers a priority after the worldwide caregiver protests of 2037. Back then, families, caregivers, nurses, and elders took to the streets by the millions to protest the lack of care options. There were mass gatherings in New York City, Kansas City, Tokyo, Barcelona, London, Mexico City, Berlin, and Moscow, among others. This lasted for almost a year. In the United States, Medicaid, Social Security, and Medicare funds had been diverted to other uses for decades, resulting in Congress moving to close the programs in the early

2030s. During this backward time, elder care was available only to the very wealthy. This is currently regarded as one of the most foolish, irresponsible, and shortsighted government mistakes in our history. Caregivers finally hit their breaking point and stood up for the needs and rights of the people they loved, making life better for all of us.

The global nurse shortage reached 65 percent in 2035. This resulted in hospitals and nursing homes becoming overloaded and eventually led to closings around the world. Outdated immigration laws in the United States, Russia, and Great Britain caused the problem to worsen due to an additional 85 percent shortage of certified nurse assistants and direct-care staff. These countries saw a third of their hospitals and almost half of their nursing homes and assisted living homes close within a ten-year period. This created a massive recession due to families leaving the workforce to provide care. Consumer spending dropped by over 40 percent throughout the developed world as families were forced to divert the majority of their income to care. These facility closings also created a housing crisis for seniors, causing homelessness among seniors to skyrocket. Families, elders, and professional caregivers joined together to push for medical advances in dementia research and for more care options.

In 2037, dementia medications were still limited to Aricept, Exelon, Razadyne, Namzaric, and Namenda. No real progress in medical research had been made in more than twenty years, creating a modern Dark Age. For decades, funding for research had failed to keep up with the severity of the problem. By the end of the 2030s, this long lack of attention had turned into a global crisis.

By 2038, the United Nations declared that providing care for elders and finding a cure for progressive dementia would become worldwide priorities for the next century. Most major governments followed suit. Caregiving became priority No. 1 in response to the chaos that decades of ignoring elders and families had created. Countries such as Peru, Mexico, Brazil, and Mali seized on this global crisis, working to rebuild their economies by doing drug research and training nurses and caregivers for the global market. The Miraflores Nursing and Medicine Cooperative, based in Lima, Peru, became the most profitable corporation in the world by 2047. Founded by a group of four women who were all caregivers, this corporation has remained in the top five ever since. By fusing care with medical research, some sensible and affordable alternatives have been created, and considerable profits made.

Now, forty years after the crisis, life is better.

Medications and caregiving

Forgive me for this little drift into science fiction, but many parts of this scenario are based on current trends in research, demographics, and current debates on healthcare policy. We have made minimal progress over the past twenty years in finding medical interventions for progressive dementia. Our current funding levels for research do not come anywhere near what should be allotted for the sixth leading cause of death in the United States. Despite recent moderate increases in funding for research, the medications that address progressive dementia are limited, and funding for care has not been increased.

Funding for care is likely to become an intense political battle in the next ten or more years. This will affect how medications are used for better or worse. When caregivers lack good support and options, medications end up being used to fill the gap. This does not work. Medications for progressive dementia are an odd combination of limited, comforting, somewhat helpful, complex, and at times irritating. Now and then, they can make life much, much better. Sometimes these medications may help keep an elder more mentally present for a few more years. But medications do not exist or work in a void. As Dr. G. Allen Power has clearly pointed out in his writing, medications do not solve the problems of well-being. Medications also do not solve the problems of caregiver fatigue, guilt, or burnout. Often, medications can be a symptom of these three problems.

That said, we have made progress. There is much less of an Alzheimer's "closet" than when I began working with the disease. We talk about dementia in public now. Therapeutic interventions such as art, music, poetry, and dance have left the category of "alternative" and are being embraced as mainstream interventions. The discussion around medication has become more nuanced. There is some good, solid research being committed to nutrition, supplements, Oriental medicine, bodywork, and herbal remedies as supportive therapy for progressive dementia.

However, there are also some slick scam artists out there. All interventions should be discussed with a doctor; interactions, especially with herbs and supplements, can be complex.

While there is no miracle out there, some bright spots are emerging. We are beginning to expect and demand good, loving care. That has not always been the case. The institutional stereotype is also being challenged. My hope is that at some point in the future, the care first/love rules approach that Vista Living Care has fostered for twenty years becomes the norm, not the exception.

Important questions

I know that this is a roundabout way into medication. But medication is never a stand-alone issue. There are always many factors to consider: Where is someone in the disease process? What is the elder's health history? Do they have issues such as irritable bowel syndrome or low blood pressure that may affect their ability to tolerate the medications for memory loss? How do both the elder and the family feel about accepting or attempting to slow the progression of the disease—is there agreement or disagreement around these issues within the family? Is the elder in end-of-life? Is polypharmacy a potential problem? What issues do they have around finances and health insurance? Is medication being used as an expression of a family member's guilt and not for the benefit of the elder? Are there issues with substance abuse? Is there a history of clinical depression or PTSD? Will the elder be reasonably compliant with a medication routine?

After all the questions, the medications for dementia fall into a few basic categories.

Cholinesterase inhibitors

The backbone of dementia medication is the cholinesterase inhibitors. These medications, including Aricept, Razadyne, and Exelon, prevent or reduce the breakdown of acetylcholine in the brain, freeing up more of this neurotransmitter to pass messages in the brain. The more neurons that are awake and passing messages, the slower the brain dies. (Aricept and Razadyne come in pill form; Exelon comes in both pills and transdermal patches.)

Doctors disagree as to how effective these medications are and how long they should be used. The Alzheimer's Association website, among others, states that on average, these medications delay the worsening of symptoms from six and twelve months. However, doctors I have worked with have given a range of one to three years. These medications are generally more effective in the earlier stages, but how long they should be taken is debated. Some doctors feel strongly that if these medications are discontinued, an elder will decline at a more rapid pace; others disagree.

As a caregiver, the questions at some point become, What are we preserving? Is this medication actually making the person's life more comfortable? In my experience, when these medications are discontinued, I have seen severe drops in only two elders. More frequently I have seen minor drops in verbal skills, coordination, and attention span. (This is purely observation and not clinical research.) I have also frequently seen the scenario of an elder going on palliative care because the family and physician decided to stop fighting the disease medically. After the majority of their medications are stopped, the elder will often feel better and be more relaxed, or have more energy and be more comfortable. Quality of life and duration of life are not the same thing.

The side effects to these medications can include nausea, vomiting, decreased appetite, increased bowel movements, loose stools, fatigue, dizziness, increased urination, nervousness, and confusion. (Exelon in patch form frequently causes a drop in blood pressure.) The problem with these side effects is that they can mimic or increase issues that can also be part of progressive dementia, such as loss of appetite, fatigue, confusion, and decreased blood pressure. Dr. Toni Camp once jokingly told me that everyone who could not tolerate Exelon ended up at Vista. While this is an exaggeration, we do frequently see people who have issues with side effects. According to the *Prescribers' Digital Reference*, cholinesterase inhibitors should be used with caution in people with gastrointestinal issues as they may cause "mild and transient" nausea, vomiting, and diarrhea. The standard protocol for starting these medications is to begin with a low dose and gradually increase to a therapeutic level over several weeks.

Glutamate regulators

The other medication that is currently a mainstay of dementia care is Namenda. Unlike Aricept and Exelon, Namenda is effective throughout the dementia process. This medication regulates glutamate, an important brain chemical. In many people with mid- to late-stage dementia, the brain overproduces this chemical; Namenda decreases that overproduction.

It is most commonly used with Aricept or Exelon, creating what is called the "Alzheimer's cocktail." The combination of these medications can be an effective approach because they affect the brain differently, thus improving the results of each other. While this is not a cure, it is widely considered to be moderately helpful. The goal of this treatment is to preserve functional ability.

The side effects of Namenda are mixed. There is potential for diarrhea or constipation, headaches, dizziness, anxiety, and one rather strange and somewhat rare side effect—nightmares that create confusion upon waking. An odd note is that an elder may tolerate this medication well initially only to develop side effects after being on it for years.

An elder living at Vista had used Namenda for more than two years when her caregivers started noticing that she was having a hard time sleeping and would awaken tearful, angry, and frightened. Prior to this she had been sleeping pretty well and was confused, but not angry or fearful. The doctor ordered the staff to check for a urinary infection, but there was none. The caregivers tried quiet music, a nightlight, warm milk, and praying the rosary with her, but the sleep problems got worse. The lady became convinced that the caregivers were worshipping Satan in the living room and that he lived there. Of course, they were not, and he did not.

Our nurse looked up each of the elder's medications for side effects and found that nightmares and extreme anxiety were rare side effects. The elder's nephew, her doctor, and our staff agreed to try stopping the Namenda rather than adding behavior medication. This ended up being a wise choice. The nightmares stopped within a week. She did have a harder time completing sentences after stopping this medicine, but Satan moved out of our living room. Her life was better and happier without Namenda. This is a rare response, but it is useful to remember that the elder whom one is caring for could be that one person in a million who responds to a medication in a bizarre way. Recall my reference to snowflakes and how individual each elder truly is.

Namzaric is a combination of Namenda and Aricept in one extended-release pill. It came on the U.S. market in 2016. It has side effects similar to both Namenda and Aricept. Because it is so new, long-term studies are not available.

Additional medications

Other forms of medication include non-steroidal anti-inflammatory drugs (NSAIDS), blood thinners, anti-depressants, anti-psychotics, anti-seizure medications, and anti-anxiety medications. Also frequently used are vitamins C, B6, B12, and E; herbal remedies; and supplements such as fish oil, CoQ10, and coconut oil. Many of these medications are used to calm symptoms of dementia or to relieve behavioral issues. Dr. G. Allen Power, who is part of the Eden Alternative movement, has done a considerable amount of writing about the use of behavioral medications with elderly dementia patients. He brings up excellent points about respecting every elder and accepting their "right to feel." Medication cannot solve the problems of dementia—these problems may be masked or quieted, but they do not disappear. The balance to all of this is comfort. Is the elder feeling more secure in their own skin with a medication or not? Are they better able to live life with or without it? Being asleep is not feeling comfortable in one's own skin. Neither is having so much internal chaos that they can't tolerate the world around them.

The other question that needs to be asked is, Who is this really for? This question applies to both families and facilities, and not only to behavioral medications. I have seen people on hospice who are still being pushed to take vitamins, supplements, and a full range of other medications even though it creates stress every day. Those vitamins could have more to do with the unresolved feelings of family members than an elder's health and comfort.

It can be hard as a caregiver in any capacity to know where the person you are caring for ends and you begin. To allow another person to have a good and comfortable life, especially someone you love, you have to be clear about this. Many elders, as well as other terminally ill people, get to a point in their lives where they just do not want to take any more medications than they absolutely have to. The first place most of us go is to try every way we can to change the form of the medication by hiding it in food, switching to patches and creams, or resorting to other creative and occasionally desperate ways to sneak medicine into someone. This may work for a while, but it will not work forever. Often the answer is to stop pushing against the current. It becomes a matter of allowing yourself as caregiver to trust the instincts of the person you are caring for.

Even in the deepest stages of dementia or illness, there is an unconscious part of the person that knows what they need to feel comfortable. My brother Morgan went through this in August of 2017. He just decided to stop taking most of his medicine, and his doctor agreed with his decision. All of the odds and ends were stopped. The end result is that he feels better on three pills a day than he did on eight. His blood pressure is very low and he does sleep more, but he eats a little better. We no longer struggle with pills every morning. He starts the day happy.

Medications for behavior or comfort

This brings us to the "anti-" medications. Anti-depressants such as Zoloft, Lexapro, and Remeron are frequently given to elders facing dementia. The primary reason for this is to help them cope with the changes they are going through and to soften the often intense emotions that can come from living with progressive dementia. These drugs can be a comfort measure, but they do not create miracles. Another use for anti-depressants is actually to take advantage of the side effects. Some of these medications have side effects such as improved sleep, increased eating, weight gain, and other effects that can be used to balance out either disease progression or problems with memory medications.

Anti-anxiety and anti-psychotic medications are tricky—they fall into the category of mixed blessings. Elders facing progressive dementia may need to have these medications changed frequently. It may not be the best idea to have them on the ninety-day supply discount plan. For some elders, these medications can allow them to live in their own skin and feel comfortable; for others, they are a disaster. Consulting a neurologist or psychiatrist is useful if behavioral issues are causing discomfort or creating unsafe situations. As Dr. Power points out so well, medication cannot take the place of well-being. Side effects can be an issue as well. There is an increased risk for falls, fatigue, changes in appetite, cardiac issues, and confusion.

Caution and comfort are the watchwords when considering these medications.

Risk factors

Medications for Lewy body dementias pose two major risks: the "paradoxical effect" and "neuroleptic malignancy syndrome," or NMS. Paradoxical effect is the phenomenon of a medication having the opposite effect than what it is given for. An anti-anxiety medication can speed someone up, raise anxiety levels, and increase blood pressure; an anti-psychotic can increase aggressive behaviors and hallucinations. This response can also occur in people with frontotemporal dementia, EtOH dementia, and people with Down syndrome who are also facing Alzheimer's disease.

NMS is a very serious reaction to a certain family of antipsychotic medications that can cause fever, muscle weakness or stiffness, poor balance, and unstable blood pressure. This reaction is life threatening and should be addressed immediately. Elders facing Lewy body dementia are highly susceptible to this. Elders facing frontotemporal dementia may also be affected.

Anti-seizure medication and dementia

Anti-seizure medications such as Depakote may also be used for people with dementia. Some elders do develop seizure activity; for others, these medications may be used instead of anti-psychotics to decrease behavioral issues and allow them to have some comfort in their own skin. The primary side effect is over-sedation. Because some elders become very sleepy with these medications, starting with a low dose and gradually increasing if needed is important. As with the other "anti-" medications, they do not suddenly make someone comfortable, happy, or safe. For some elders, they may allow a bit of comfort if approach, environment, attention, and care have not provided enough comfort. But no medication can ever take the place of care or love.

Sometimes these medications are used in an attempt to keep an elder safe in an environment that no longer suits their level of confusion. Changing the environment is often a more positive solution than trying to medicate elders to fit in a place that no longer meets their needs. Honesty and an ethical core are important here. The toughest and most important thing for any caregiver, family, or professional to be aware of is what they cannot do. I encourage people to be honest even if it hurts. And it will hurt. Sometimes love is not enough. Sometimes an elder will need a different kind of structure and care. If this is true, medication can't fix that. No medication can make someone not have dementia. No medication can make an elder or caregiver safe.

NSAIDS and pain medications

Anti-inflammatory medications are used as a comfort measure for many elders with or without dementia for aches and pains. However, they do pose a risk for stomach irritation and some can have the effect of thinning the blood. Some elders also use stronger pain relievers, including opioids, which can increase confusion, fall risk, and fatigue. Pain issues with dementia can be complicated. There is often a concern that an elder with mid- to late-stage dementia will under-report pain. I have also rather frequently seen elders who are over-prescribed pain medications. This is common in elders who are trying to live in an environment that is not suited to dementia.

Often an elder will be more willing to move their body in a place that feels safe, and increased mobility often means less pain. Having other people to talk to who don't care if you repeat yourself is a good distraction from a sore back. Depression feeds pain; security and love decrease pain. At Vista Living Care, we have elders whose pain medications have been reduced or discontinued because much of the pain they were reporting was really confusion and sadness.

Looking for a miracle in a bottle

Vitamins, herbal medicines, and supplements are probably much more useful for caregivers who need to preserve their own health, energy, and immune systems than for someone with mid- to late-stage dementia. There is a mindboggling amount of information out there on these substances; some of the studies are excellent and some are just glorified marketing campaigns. Be careful of looking for a miracle in a bottle. There isn't one.

The film and advertising industries often oversimplify, romanticize, or disregard the need for elders and caregivers to have honest, informed images of their lives. Our society alternates between what Eden Alternative calls the "tragedy narrative" and the "my husband, wife, mother, or father could hardly speak, walk, or feed themselves, and now after taking fill-in-the-blank or changing their diet or you name it, they are driving, dancing, and balancing the checkbook" infomercials. These false images do not help elders or their families. What we need is a true image of how complex life really is for elders and caregivers. While there is no miracle cure to make dementia go away, there are still light and joy in the face of disease. People do not live in complete tragedy or victimhood. People also do not suddenly get better.

Taking complex protocols of pills, drinks, and specialized foods can be a major issue for someone with dementia. My question is, Does this create comfort or joy? There is some really fascinating and hopeful research into how supplements, herbs, and vitamins can clean up plaques in the brain and improve life with dementia. Then the question becomes, Can an elder follow the routine, even with help from a caregiver? Is actually getting the food, pills, or shakes into the elder a daily struggle?

Progressive dementia is currently fatal. This does not mean that an elder who is facing any of these illnesses should not have the most healthy, joyful, and loving life possible. But that does not come from a bottle. Often it means making life simpler. The poet Maya Angelou writes, "Poetry is the process of eliminating words." Caring for someone with dementia can be like this. All parts of life should become more pure, more essential; the things that are not comforting should at some point go away. This applies to any medicine, vitamin, or treatment. If it is making life more frustrating or confusing, no matter how good it is supposed to be for the body or brain, it should be eliminated. Life is to be lived, not maintained with pills.

Hero Stories

Our teachers, our heroes

I hate the word victim. The elders whom I have been blessed to meet over the past twenty years are many things, but they are not victims. They are fighting a battle that they will not win. They face an illness that will at some point likely kill them. But I have never met anyone facing dementia who did not find some way to stand strong against this process, to be human, connected, creative, loving, funny, and alive in spite of it all. I have not met victims. I have met fighters and friends, the most stubborn, tough—and yes, fragile—human beings on the planet. None of them gave up. All of them found ways to be truly, deeply human. Our Vista Living Care community is deeply blessed by our elders. In the heroism of their struggle, they make our town a better place to live.

My brother needs some kind of care each day. He also rises above difficulty with grace, humor, and toughness. He sings his own mean versions of "The Lion Sleeps Tonight," "Welcome to the Jungle," and "Stairway to Heaven." Morgan also paints, babysits, and cares for our two pets, Flor the cat and Honey the dog. Each day is an adventure despite the complications of Down syndrome and heart failure. Every day he fights fiercely to live, and on many days he fights to breathe. He still loves the life that he has been given. Needing help and care are simply a part of his life, not the definition of his life. Morgan and the elders who face dementia show all of us how to be brave, how to love, how to find joy in life. They are infinite sources of inspiration. Respect for each individual who needs help allows more room for freedom for all involved. Ultimately, it makes care easier and more free.

Every day Jeanne gets up. Every day she fights to walk. Every day she holds someone's hand. Every day she laughs. Now and then, she forgets how to swallow. She has stood against an enemy inside her for seven years now. That enemy has taken her words. In the face of that enemy, Jeanne fell deeply, passionately, devotedly in love. Now she sees a world that the people around her don't get to witness. Now her life and presence are melting into pure kindness. Everyone is blessed with her smile, her hugs, and her giggle. In spite of the enemy in her brain, she has made paintings and has lived gracefully.

We met Sherry one Saturday because she tried to climb out a second-story window. She used to be an English professor. We believe she was the one the freshmen were all afraid of. She seldom speaks, but when she does, you are usually in trouble. She is decisive; she does not waffle or hesitate. Without words, she is still crystal clear about what she wants and does not want. "No" means it's not going to happen; give it up. She baffles doctors; I think she enjoys that. Her body stopped cooperating with her a long time ago, but she keeps going. She beats the odds every day. She is tough. She is beautiful. She commands attention. She will not tolerate nonsense. She loves her men. She is a kind friend. She senses loyalty. Sherry is a hero.

Frankie sang all the time, for years, almost any song you could think of. She knew all the gospel songs and all the drinking songs. After a while the lyrics got a bit odd, but she sang anyway. Frankie was a loyal friend. She could be demanding and a bit of a princess at times. Aren't we all? Every man she met just adored her. (I wish I could pull that one off.) I came down the hall one day to find her singing "A Hundred Bottles of Beer on the Wall" at the top of her lungs with our local priest. They were both laughing.

Frankie always tried to do everything except for exercise. Eye rolling was her favorite physical activity. She was always the first to arrive to a party and usually the last to leave. She always sat closest to the band. She taught us that chocolate is the most important food group. When talking to anyone, she began with, "I like you, I love you"—a good place to start any discussion, even when she disagreed with the other person. She believed in speaking her mind and did so with charm. She was always proud of her children. They somehow became the perfect kids as she got older. Hair and makeup were appreciated; manicures were not. Frankie met the last nine years of Alzheimer's on her own terms. Her terms were music, stubbornness, friendship, and as much chocolate as possible.

For more than a year, Joan drew every day. Hundreds and hundreds of pages of spirals, webs of subtle color making mysterious worlds. These drawings became her novel, her obsession, her home. She created a world to go to when words failed her, a world that could often become obsessive, spilling out onto walls, bed sheets, and pillowcases. Our caregivers and her family made sure she had really good tools to work with. We would set her up with materials, remind her to take breaks, and offer snacks and drinks that allowed her to stay strong. We learned that she would forget to eat or drink, that she needed help coming out of this world she had created. Our staff created the structure that her brain could not. By giving her the structure she needed and helping her stay strong, we were rewarded by getting to see her new drawings, in pencil, ink, and watercolor.

Joan and her husband agreed to share her journals in Alzheimer's education talks. The students see her work and are amazed; they smile and then they cry. They learn that life with dementia is much more complicated and beautiful than they could have imagined. She and I sit and look at other artists' work in books—Paul Klee, Georgia O'Keeffe, Leonardo DaVinci. She likes Klee and DaVinci, but thinks O'Keeffe is "too simple, kind of sleepy." Some of her drawings remind me of DaVinci's flood drawings, the intricate, twisting lines and spirals showing what it feels like to be drowning. She draws beauty, humor, and pain. She is an artist; this is her work. Today she looks more and draws less. She rests more now. She gets scared often, but she keeps going. Each day she keeps up the fight, with color and line. Each day she loses a little. Joan is a hero.

Family stories

The fight against dementia is by nature a shared effort. Elders facing dementia live, create, love, laugh, and explore in the midst of a dying brain. Families, husbands, wives, daughters, sons, friends are drawn in to share the challenge. They carry the memories that the person they love is losing. They bear the weight of the past and hold all that could have been. Families and friends know what is being lost, both the good and the bad. But the elder at some point gets to forget; they get to melt into the eternal present.

Over the years, like all the caregivers at Vista, I have been present with elders in their dementia. I have seen their losses and their victories, but I do not carry their past. I did not know the lawyer who had mastered words and turned those words into power; I dance with a man who is charming and friendly and devoted to his lady friend. I did not know the woman who tried to disown her daughter for wanting to be an artist; I painted with an amazing woman, and one of her paintings hangs in my living room today. I never met the man who wrote speeches for my father's favorite president, or the man who walked out on his family; I got to know the man who sang beautifully and told dirty jokes that would peel the paint off the walls—some complicated and rather graphic storytelling on his part turned "Yankee Doodle Dandy" into a tale of unplanned pregnancy and shotguns. We don't carry the loss in the same way. We don't carry the love or the anger, the baggage.

A friend of mine, we'll call her Bobbi, saw her mother through Lewy body disease. Before dementia she used to refer to her mother as "Mommy Dearest" with utmost sarcasm. Mom had been abusive in many ways throughout her life, to everyone around her. Dementia did not change her mother's basic personality. Instead of being a mean and very organized lady, Mom became a mean and very confused lady. In honor of her father, my friend managed her mother's care. She realized early on that she could not do the hands-on care, so she chose the most loving option. Bobbi carefully managed the family finances and found great people to care for her mom. When it became impossible to care for Mom at home, she sought out assisted living.

Mom had anger issues both from her personality and the disease process. Mom knew how to insult and demean caregivers even after she lost the ability to speak. By then it was just who she was; the person and the disease had merged. Neither approach nor medication would change that. Bobbi was a great support to the staff and always expressed gratitude for her mom's care. I got many calls from her during this time. She learned about the disease through our long distance calls and stayed in close touch with her mom's caregivers. Mom ended up with the best life that she herself would allow. Her daughter ended up feeling calm, and a sense of closure. She had done the right thing. She had been responsible, and she had shown respect.

Bobbi has been a teacher for me in some very important ways. She taught me that it can be heroic to know your own boundaries. She taught me that it can be loving to know when to let go. In making the decision to set up her mother's care in a sensible, respectful, and considerate way, Bobbi was able to release the ghosts of the past. Too often we tend to look at caregiving in terms of how much is sacrificed. But stress and fatigue are not measures of how loving we are. Often, adult children and spouses—especially spouses—carry the belief that if they are not doing the hands-on care, despite whatever issues the past presents, they are failing. This is not true.

In the face of life threatening illness there are many, many ways to be a hero. The partner who stands by their mate and supports both freedom and comfort, even when they struggle with or do not want to see the changes their partner is going through, is a hero. The ex-wife who takes her dementia-suffering former husband into her home when everyone else has turned their backs on him is a hero. The husband who cares lovingly for his wife at home is a hero. So is the husband who finds the home where his wife can be a social butterfly. Yes, there is fear, sadness, and frustration. But they keep going.

The daughter who was the family peacemaker and lost sleep trying to get the family to accept that Momma needed help is a hero. So is the daughter who raised hell, alienated her family, and pulled her parents out of a toxic situation. For years, there would be court visits and fighting, but both her parents would be safe and happy until their deaths.

The daughter who spent years crying, planning, and organizing from two thousand miles away so she could provide the home she knew her father would eventually need is a hero. The son who went to visit his mother, who sounded "great on the phone, but when I got there, it was just bad," and made the immediate decision to move his mother out of the home she had lived in for sixty-something years and across the country to be near him is a hero.

The daughter who, as she faced late-stage cancer, cared for both her mother with Alzheimer's and her brother with Down syndrome, is a hero. First this daughter cared for her mother and brother when they lived in their own homes, then in her home, and then in the facility she scraped up the money for. The ability to stand by the family she loved no matter what—

no matter how complicated, or frustrating, or how many changes were required—still gives me hope.

The seventeen-year-old granddaughter who put her college fund into keeping her grandmother in assisted living at the end of Gram-gram's life is a hero.

The book club friends who became caregivers for one of their members are heroes. They helped her stay in her home in the country for years. When this was no longer possible, they did all the paperwork, cleaning, and moving so that she would be cared for. These amazing people made the choice to stand by their friend.

They have different relationships—some are family by blood, some are partners, others are friends—but they all have made the choice to stand by someone, to do what is needed to protect someone they love. It is the act of making choices that creates our world. In my work with dementia at Vista Living Care, I am blessed to see how many good people there are out there. These choices show how brave, strong, and decent we as human beings can be. These people do not always make the same choice, but they make choices for the same reasons: love, respect, and honor. This is what matters.

Respect

Professional caregivers in their many forms also make daily choices to love. They have made a commitment to do whatever they can to help. They do really difficult and often unpleasant work. I admit that I have a bias here. I have worked for more than twenty years with CNAs, direct-care staff, and home caregivers, and I am protective of them. Over the years I have seen firsthand how unfair and relentless the criticism can be toward facility caregivers and, to a lesser extent, home health workers. I have also been blessed to work with many, many families who really understand how hard these caregivers work and support what they do.

That said, we have a problem in this country with how we view the profession of caregiving. This problem often comes from other professionals. The lawyer ads that imply that all nursing and assisted-living homes are staffed with people who are just there to abuse elders and collect a paycheck are one face of this. The consultant who wants to "fix" the CNAs without looking at the system they work in is another. The doctors, social workers, and case managers who automatically assume that elders will be ignored or neglected in care facilities are another. There are professionals out there who believe the observations of direct-care staff are "the lowest form of information"—yes, I know of a doctor who actually said this. That statement still gives me nightmares.

These people are all major contributors to this problem, adding more stress and fatigue to the lives of everyone involved. These attitudes only open the door for burnout. They increase the turnover in a field that requires skill and commitment. If we really want to improve care in this country, we need to begin by respecting the hardworking people who do the day-in, day-out hands-on care. Without this basic respect, all other changes are just window dressing that will do little to improve the lives of elders and families. At Vista Living, our direct-care staff are the heartbeat of our homes. They are closest to our elders, and their observations are often the most relevant.

The snowstorm of 2006

I had the privilege of being part of the Vista Living Care family during the biggest winter storm in Santa Fe's history. It was New Year's weekend, 2006, when we got more than three feet of snow. I was on call, but snowed in at home. (Santa Fe is notoriously poor at snow removal—three feet of snow means nothing moves on the roads.) But our elders were well cared for because of the devotion of our caregivers and nurse, Shelia. Two caregivers walked to work from their apartment complex, which was about a mile away. Shelia moved in for three days. Another caregiver, whose husband was stranded at work out of town, moved in with her two children. I kept the phones transferred to my house and became the switchboard for the better part of three days.

They all ate together, spent time with the elders, played games, did manicures, made popcorn, baked cookies, watched old movies, and cleaned house. When we all got back to work, we arrived at an orderly, beautiful home filled with happy elders. One of our elders described it as a "slumber party with snow." On top of all that success, there was very little overtime pay. The caregivers had worked out downtime with one another and traded shifts brilliantly. We were out of popcorn and chocolate chips, and all of the ladies sported fresh colorful nails. This is one small example of caregiver intelligence, creativity, responsibility, and heroism. These ladies took ownership of the home they worked in and made the choice to stand with their elders because they were family.

Teaching life

I see caregivers doing kind, loving acts each day. I have seen them patiently deal with being hit, kicked, spat on, and called names. (Recently, a ninety-eight-year old who weighed about ninety pounds clocked a caregiver and broke her nose.) And I have also seen them receive love and become family to many elders. Through the work they do, they also become teachers for our elders in many ways.

Several years ago, when I was teaching an art class at a senior center, I worked with an elder who was raised in South Texas during the time of segregation. She still held much of the bias she had grown up with and frequently expressed her views. When her dementia worsened, she moved into Vista where she developed a deep trust and friendship with the caregivers. These amazing ladies were from Mexico and Central

America. One day, when this lady was in Walmart with her daughter, she saw a caregiver with whom she had become close and broke away from her daughter to give the caregiver a huge hug and kiss. The woman's daughter was not comfortable with her mother being publicly affectionate with one of "those people." It became clear that while the mother had grown as a person, the daughter had not. It was painful for the caregiver, but the coldness of the family never changed the caregiver's love for the elder. The elder's caregivers were her guides to a more free and loving life.

Thank you, I love you

There are so many stories around caregiving, but in truth the most important story is about relationship, love, and gratitude. This story started with a ringing telephone in the middle of the night.

Two caregivers stepped into a dim room. A whispering voice said, "Come here." One caregiver sat on the bed next to a very thin, very frail, elderly lady who had barely spoken in years. The other caregiver stood near the head of the bed. The lady breathed deeply, and in a clear, strong voice said, "Thank you. I love you." She then took a soft breath, closed her eyes, and stopped breathing.

These final words were the expression of a deep connection between an elder and her caregivers. The last words of this woman's life were a testament to just how meaningful her relationship was with the women who had helped her with day-to-day life at Vista. So much is made about what is lost with dementia that we often forget how elders can ultimately live in innocence, clarity, and enlightenment. We forget the bond between elder and caregiver. I can only hope that my own last words will be, "Thank you, I love you."

Myths About Dementia Care

There are many myths out there regarding dementia and caregiving. From the perspective of watching families struggle with this, I have compiled a list about the misconceptions and unproductive responses that get in the way of care and make life tougher for everyone involved. Myths can be comforting, but they can also be limiting and unkind. They prevent families from seeing what is right in front of them.

Myth #1: Home is always better.

Is home always better? The "always" is the problem here. Many elders with dementia find their lives become very restricted in a house or apartment that they can no longer manage. Some who have the means may have round-the-clock caregivers just an arm's length away, which means a loss of privacy. Certain safety and ethical issues such as wandering, pica, medication management, disrupted sleep, and other changes can be far more difficult to deal with in a home setting, especially if the primary caregiver is sharing the home. We have also seen a variety of in-home caregivers and agencies exploit struggling families for monetary gain. Often the companionship of peers, daily professional interaction, ongoing assessments for inevitable changes, and social stimulation give elders a sense of freedom they otherwise would not have in a home setting.

I remember doing an evaluation several years ago. The gentleman was angry, yelling, and striking out at his wife and caregivers. I took a short walk with him and asked him how he felt. He gave a one-word answer: "Henpecked!" He spent his days with amazing women who tended to him beautifully and did everything humanly possible to keep him safe. The only thing he lacked in his life was freedom. His home was lovely, immaculate, but not functional for him without constant assistance. He simply could not get space from his caregivers, ever—a caregiver even stayed in his room at night to prevent falls. This man was loved and well cared for, but the constant, unrelenting love and care he received had become an irritant.

One of our lovely elders lived independently in a large, beautiful assisted-living apartment for several years. But as she became more confused, she was no longer welcomed by her more "functional" peers. She became depressed, was not eating well, and was fearful of leaving her apartment. Her doctor advised hospice. (Our industry has unfortunately seen a spike in hospice admissions due in part to independent living facilities retaining elders longer than is appropriate.) Her daughter did some research, opted out of hospice, and went with Vista Living Care instead.

The woman blossomed. She needed the company of people who repeated themselves, and who accepted her for who she was. In a house for dementia, her world got much bigger. She found community. She found she could express her somewhat warped sense of humor, her love of animals, and her deep affection for people without limits or judgment. She could be the person she really was. In getting care and help, she became far more independent. Her daughter did not take anything away from her mother by moving her to a "dementia facility." She gave her mother the gift of friendships that would endure to the end of her life. Yes, she struggled, and dementia eventually took her life. But for a time there was joy, love, laughter, and peace of mind for both family and elder.

Home is the right choice for some people. Large, beautiful independent-living apartments can be wonderful, but not for everyone. For many, their needs will change during the aging process with or without dementia. As caregivers, we need to be open-minded enough to see beyond the myths, misplaced promises, and fears that stand in the way. We need to remember that we are part of the equation and work to find a situation that works for both elder and caregiver.

Many families make promises such as, "I will never put you away in one of those places." But in progressive dementia, our promises mean little. There is an obvious and vast difference between a really good life before dementia and a really good life after dementia. Common knowledge tells us that life changes, which applies to care placement as well. We have to find ways to adjust with elders as they change. We have learned to be responsive to the needs of people with other life changing illnesses such as cancer and HIV. This responsive approach has made life better for people facing these illnesses. We now need to become more responsive to Alzheimer's and dementia care and the ever-changing needs of elders.

Myth #2: My loved one is "not like those people."

When I was a kid in church, our pastor would talk about "that still small voice," meaning we had to be open enough to hear or see a way through any problem by paying attention to spirit. Caregivers often become so busy facing each day that it is hard to be quiet long enough to hear, feel, or see what the heart and spirit have to say. My father, a single parent who was widowed when we were young, put this in a tougher way. He would say, "God will speak in the still small voice until he gets tired of you not listening, and then he will kick you in the backside." What he meant is that sooner or later, if we did not pay attention, a problem would catch up with us and become a crisis.

The notion that a loved one is "not like those people" and "not that confused" gets in the way of families getting the right support at the right time. Often people want to believe this myth until a crisis develops. I have seen families second-guess themselves and opt for denial only to end up with a health or safety crisis weeks, days, or even hours later. Trust your instincts. If you sense that there is a problem, you are usually right. Don't let the crisis make the decision rather than your family. Options such as going on a wait list for assisted living placement or for community services can evaporate because suddenly something has to be done NOW. That can end up meaning you take what you can get instead of choosing what you want for the person you are caring for. Yes, the person you love may not be that con-fused today, but in six months or six weeks, things could be very different. Prepare for a future you can't predict.

If you visit a place that you think the person you are caring for would be happy in, or you find a type of care that your elder will likely need at some point, get on the wait list. Even if you think you may not need it or that everything is going well at home, prepare for that unpredictable future. If you are facing the need for Medicaid or VA services, this is even more im-portant. There will be wait lists; it all takes time. Getting ap-plications completed that may take years to process is critical, even if the person you love is doing well now. Start early and be tenacious. Common sense and planning can be a loving and spiritual process. Caregivers who allow themselves to truly *see* the person they are caring for and *see* their needs express a deep form of love.

Myth #3: If only we had more and better interventions, our elder would get better.

"If my dad were more active, if we try a different medica-tion, if he takes fish oil, if he becomes a vegan, if we go to church more, if we attend more concerts, if we see a better doctor or go to a better clinic, if I pray more, if I were there more often, if I bring lunch to the facility...*if I do more, Dad will get better.*"

The "more/better" myth, or the "toxic ifs," cloud a caregiver's vision. It is normal, human, and loving to want to make life better for someone you care for. The problem is that sometimes we push people we love so hard to be healthy, active, or normal that we wear out both them and ourselves. Guilt lives here, as do bargaining and denial, and guilt is easily shared. The home health aide or the activities director or caregiver in the facility is not going to start walking on water just because you promised your parents that they could stay in their house but then found out they could not. All any of us can do is be honest, present, and loving, and keep standing by someone as they change.

There is a rather large industry out there that promotes supplements, diet, treatments, and herbal medicine to help with dementia. While continued research is good, much of this falls into the more/better myth. It can become expensive, overwhelming to keep up with, and a source of guilt for families. The search for a solution to a terminal illness can keep a caregiver from what is most important, which is simply being present. There has to be a point for all of us as caregivers when we just accept that we are doing the best we possibly can. That this is as good as it gets.

It is natural to look for a miracle when caring for someone who is losing the fight against any progressive illness. And caregivers do get miracles, but mostly small ones. Many caregivers, especially family caregivers, want the huge miracle of the disease to go away so much that they don't allow themselves to really feel or see the smaller miracles, the quiet moments of grace and freedom. The laughter, the smile, the holding hands, the beautiful drawing, the healing animal, a few extra steps walking—all of these things are miracles; each one is a stand against dementia. The more/better myth gets in the way of seeing these small miracles. It is hard to connect with someone when guilt and regret are calling the shots. The incessant noise of the toxic ifs drowns out that quiet, miraculous voice that comes from being connected in love.

Myth #4: So-and-so is not doing enough.

"The doctor, the staff, my siblings, my parents, my neighbor, my pastor are simply not doing enough." The myth that someone is Not Doing Enough if dementia gets worse is closely related to the more/better and the toxic ifs myth. In reality, the loved one is usually much worse than perceived.

It is normal to be angry when we see a disease that we have known about for over a century take the mind, body, and life of someone we love. But putting that anger on the backs of other people who are working really hard to help is just not useful. Guilt often gets tangled up with anger. It can be hard to know where our responses come from. Your sister or brother who has been struggling to care for Mom or Dad did not do anything to make the disease progress faster. The caregivers at the nursing home or assisted living did not make the dementia worse. This myth assigns blame and creates dangerous denial.

More activities, different food, and more medication can make life better at times; they can also create exhaustion, frustration, and discomfort. Caregivers of all stripes do what they do out of love. Like the more/better myth, the not-doing-enough myth can blind someone to changes that can be beautiful. It is hard to acknowledge that someone is more affectionate, creative, or funny when we are lost in anger and guilt and on the lookout for someone to blame. If we view someone with dementia as nothing more than a set of losses, they cease to be a human being. This does not mean that the losses are not there. But it also does not mean that the person you love isn't "still in there."

Myth #5: The family can handle this with simple, logical solutions.

When trapped in the "simplified reality" myth, we may oversimplify a problem or react without being aware of the reasoning behind our actions. Some people will find any reason to procrastinate when a decision is needed, and avoidance and denial are common responses: "We have plenty of time. We can wait to make these plans. We're fine." An elder's condition may also be minimized: "Mom only wandered away, or fell, or bounced a check, or missed a meal, or skipped her medications once—it won't happen again." Terminal illness is always a crisis, but dementia makes this crisis more complex and long lasting. Dementia can be easier to hide from, deny, or lie to yourself and others about than, say, bronchitis.

Some people become overly logical to deny their own feelings. Family members can also become trapped in the roles of placator, blamer, or distracter. The decision-maker may think, "I'll do something when I can get the whole family to agree," or "I don't want to upset my brother or sister," or "I don't want Mom or Dad to be mad at me."

Every family creates its own stories, its own particular mythology about how the world works and how struggles should be faced. These stories can be kind and loving and feed the soul. They can also be mean, toxic, and disruptive. Many families do work together, learn, and grow in the face of dementia. Some do not. Sometimes an elder with dementia becomes a pawn in family discord and power struggles.

Lies and denial take time and energy that would be far better used in facing the disease and loving the person with that disease. It can take time to get families to agree on simple things like who is driving or where to meet for lunch. What to do when someone they love is struggling with seemingly simple parts of their life and needs help that they don't want is much tougher. Sometimes there just isn't the luxury of getting everyone in the family to agree on the next step.

In writing these words, I realize that in many ways I am a distant observer. My family of origin is only Morgan and me. I am the caregiver, and I make the decisions. Right or wrong, I live with the choices that are our lives. Velma and Linda, my friends and family of choice, both support the decisions I make, though always from different points of view. But Morgan's life is a democracy of two, with me making the final decisions. I remember a family we worked with asking one time if I felt lonely as a caregiver. The truth is I do not. My family of choice has been there in ways that many families of origin simply aren't. I don't deal with resistance or fighting. There is no one questioning my decisions, making judgments, or not helping. There is no one pushing a direction; it is just us. Morgan and I are able to put our life together in the way we see fit. This is a gift that I am deeply grateful for. The help I get is a blessing, not a quarrel. In many ways, it is less difficult than the struggle of getting family to agree on the next step.

Family conflicts, ghosts from the past, and power struggles are much more complicated. These take time and work to face. Family mediation, counseling, support groups, and pastoral counseling are all helpful for families. The conferences put on by the Alzheimer's Association and other senior service groups can be sources of support. But there may be things in a family's history or life that can't be fixed. This is hard for a caregiver.

Much of being a caregiver is being a protector. Taking a stand is just as much a part of love as caring is. While anger can get in the way and cloud vision, anger can also create the energy to make change. The role of protector is important. It can also be a hard role to give up once you have found safety for the person you love. Yes, there is abuse, exploitation, and neglect out there—stand against it. There is also kindness, decency, and honesty—allow it.

Myth #6: We'll never get the family to work together and make decisions.

Over the years we have seen families do amazing, heroic, beautiful caregiving. We have seen families grow closer and stronger in the care they give an elder. We have seen families work through really tough problems from the past. Much of the work we do is to support families in standing with the elders they love as they face dementia. We express this with lots of talking and time. Routine family conferences are common at Vista Living Care. We believe the more informed families are about what the person they love is facing, the better life will be for everyone. Even though this can be painful and tiring, in the end, knowing is better for our elders and families.

Mona was the matriarch of a large, complicated, creative, highly accomplished, and quirky Santa Fe family. As a child, her sisters called her Bossy Boots. Mona had been the family organizer. She was the web that kept the family connections strong. Mona's life was complex, deeply and lovingly entangled with the lives of her children, sisters, husband, and devoted private caregiver. The complexity of Mona's life did not decrease with dementia. Her daughter Lisa ended up being the one who was continually getting the band together, organizing meetings, setting and keeping boundaries, and helping create a climate that would allow the entire family to learn more than they ever wanted to know about Alzheimer's disease.

Lisa unknowingly took over Mona's role as Bossy Boots in the most graceful way possible. She survived family conferences, letting go of bucket lists, and juggling the schedules of a large family in a way that actually allowed Mona to rest and be connected to all of them. Mona's family took the time to talk, to learn about dementia, and to be there for Mona in a realistic, honest way. Sometimes it was sweet and funny; just as often it was frustrating and painful. They talked, argued, and got creative about how to be with Mona as she changed. They did not settle everything; they did not fix every wrong or suddenly become perfect or ideal. They asked questions and really listened to the answers. They accepted that sometimes there were no answers. Mona remained deeply connected to everyone in her complicated life throughout her battle with dementia.

Vista Living Care had the honor of being part of this wonderful web, to educate, support, and even create an in-house dating service that allowed Mona to remain connected to her husband even though they could no longer live under the same roof. In the end, there was peace. In the end, the band stayed together, proving it is possible. Thank you, Bossy Boots and the Band.

Myth #7: People who need help are weak and worthless.

All people facing dementia will at some point need help with major parts of their lives. The truth is that all human beings need help with major parts of their lives. Independence is often a double-edged sword. All human beings need to make choices, interact with the world around them, and have control of their lives. But much of what we give elders in the name of independence is loneliness, disconnection, and frustration.

Dr. William Thomas, founder of the Eden Alternative, talks extensively about how our Western culture has created a "cult of adulthood" that only values people who are living the fantasy of independence. If you can make money, go to work, pay bills, drive, own a home, and have a level of status in the world, you are independent and have value. If not, your value as a person is questionable. The problems with this viewpoint are many. Elders, children, homemakers, caregivers, and people like my brother and his friends all get pushed to the side and not valued for the many contributions they make to the world around them. The result is we end up with a society that is less loving, less creative, less connected, and less human.

We also end up creating unnecessary suffering by pushing people toward a false definition of what it is to be independent. If an elder is getting lost and this is faced directly by a caring community without judgment, they will be safe and have more freedom. If an elder can find confidential assistance with finances in a safe environment that does not judge or exploit them, they will experience less stress and fear. What would happen if the contribution of an elder's companionship and sense of history were given a place of value in our communities, even if they could no longer live alone? If moving to a "facility" were stripped of all the false narratives and simply considered another option, life would be far less painful for elders and families. Facilities would also benefit from having to live up to being good places to live instead of descending to the stereotype of being places to hide and die. What would happen if instead of struggling with simply trying to hold it together alone in a house or apartment, elders were offered the opportunity to explore their creative, nurturing, and spiritual parts of life?

Much of what passes for independence in the lives of elders facing dementia is an unending reminder of loss, not a celebration of their humanity. If someone can nurture children and sing, but can't drive or balance a checkbook, are they of less value? How many of us face things in our lives that we need help with? I can't fix my car or my computer. Does that change my value as a person?

The myth of "it only happened once" is connected to denial and holding on to our false definition of independence. The facts are simple: It only takes once. Wandering, not tracking medications, leaving the stove on, or losing track of credit cards all have the potential to alter the path of someone's life and cause good options to vanish. While all human beings need to face risk and have choices, we do need to protect as well. If a choice is life threatening, or can create severe pain or a health crisis, it may not be a choice. Disease process is different from choice or freedom. And in reality, the unhealthy, life-threatening behavior does not happen just once; it will happen again and again. Someday, the person will get hurt if the behavior is not addressed. These problems are not in the elder's control; they are disease progression. This is about changes in the person's brain, not about stress or particular situations. For many elders, denial is part of the disease. Dementia should not be the decision-maker.

Myth #8: We can't afford care.

Healthcare has dominated the news for years now. This section is not about politics. It is about care. Unfortunately, some of the really annoying myths that dominate our politics do work their way into caregivers' lives and create guilt, stress, and failure to access needed help. People who need help with care, either physical or financial, are not lazy, weak, irresponsible or trying to scam the system. The vast majority of family caregivers are just trying to care for someone they love. They don't have the time or energy to run scams. Needing a day program, assisted living, or nursing home for someone you love is not failure. You are not "one of those people"; most Americans need financial help with elder care.

According to the Alzheimer's Association's 2018 report, the estimated lifetime cost of care for a person living with dementia is $341,840. I have not met many people who have a spare $341,840 just sitting around waiting to be used. Most families I have known have to do serious planning and learn about options for care and its costs.

If you or the person you are caring for is blessed to have saved enough to afford private pay or have long-term care insurance for care, that's great. You will still need to plan, organize, and ask questions. You will also have more options. Learn what these options are.

If you can afford assisted living for a time but will at some point need to get your loved one qualified for Medicaid services, you are in the majority. The policy at our Vista Living Care homes is to help families figure out the next step; communicating well before you are out of funds helps us help you. If you are dealing with an assisted living that will not help you find the next step, or does not take the time to talk with you, looking at other options might be worthwhile.

If you are caring for someone who has to have Medicaid services, either community-based or institutional, don't put off applying for services. Don't wait until you are exhausted from being a caregiver without any respite to apply. This will take time, often years. It will be complicated. You will probably get rejected at least once. You may be treated badly. But don't give up. Knowledge is power; learn as much as you can about the systems you are dealing with. Read the regulations. Keep asking questions. Keep making calls. Keep showing up. Fight for what you need.

Myth #9: There's nothing we can do. There's no hope.

Giving up and acceptance are very different things. Cynical mindsets ("It's not worth it, Mom's not in there anymore anyway") are potentially toxic and are in some sense a lie. They interfere with a clear vision of how to care for someone and keep families from considering options that can improve the lives of everyone involved.

Part of the motivation behind writing this book is frustration with the unbalanced way progressive dementia is often discussed. Caregiving is complex. Elders who face dementia are complex. Everyone involved has complicated, often contradictory feelings and responses to this process. Yes, there is loss and the disease processes are awful. But there is a profound difference between facing the process with open-eyed realism and cynically giving up. While we can't cure this disease, we can make the process better in real, tangible ways. The person you love may be radically different than they were in the past, but their heart and soul are still in there.

Dementia is not purely a tragedy, nor is it a simple, happy, and confused state. It is a human process. All of the mismatched, freewheeling emotions, reactions, and contradictions that make us human are part of dementia and caregiving. The struggle is matched only by fierce love. Facing progressive dementia and caring for someone with progressive dementia means to embrace the fact that someone you love is dying. It also means celebrating the life that person still has in spite of dementia and death. This time is important. While an elder with advanced dementia may not speak or understand the world in a conscious way, every elder with dementia feels and loves. They know, maybe not in a way that would make sense to the rest of us, but they know you are there. Don't give up.

Myths around dementia tend to reinforce stereotypes that work against both elders and the ability to access care. They create barriers—to ideas, options, planning, and action—that can open the door to crisis. The myths create noise that can keep us from hearing what our hearts and spirits have to say.

Disease progression in dementia varies widely and is highly unpredictable. Looking at options for hands-on care shortly after diagnosis is a good idea. Looking at care and finances early on does not mean you have to use them right away. Finding out about benefits, setting up medical and financial power of attorney paperwork, completing applications for services, putting down wait-list deposits, and learning your state's options and regulations about long-term care is not cynical or cheap or giving up the fight. It is reality.

Holding onto these myths can create unnecessary tension for families and create an environment that makes it difficult for professional caregivers to be effective. While the myths are often believed by very loving people, the consequence is not a loving one.

Right Livelihood and Falling in Love

"Some days I wonder if I'm working because what I do just feels like joy."

All good caregiving is about falling in love. This love is not some overly sweet, simplistic, always-joyful state; it is a much harder, more honest, more unpredictable, and far more real love. Good caregiving has to be realistic. Good caregiving has to love the scary, sad, and unlovable parts of dementia. Good caregiving also has to be open enough to see the creative, kind, and funny parts of dementia.

The work that I and every one of the 4.5 million professionals in the United States who work in eldercare do can be tough, painful, exhausting work. In my experience, this is work that becomes a part of you. There is an idea in Buddhism of "right livelihood," meaning the way you make your living adds kindness, peace, justice, and compassion to the world. Good caregiving does this. Systems of care can either encourage a person to grow in kindness, peace, justice, and compassion or can prevent the expression of these fundamental aspects of humanity. I am blessed to work in an environment that nurtures my basic humanity and that of our elders.

As I've worked on this book, I've listened to the ways caregivers describe their work and their reasons for staying with it. Certain words came up over and over: honor, hope, faith, joy, and love—most of all, love.

One of our Vista caregivers put this beautifully when she

said, "I do my job with love. In the beginning, I just needed the job. Then I realized I was falling in love with these elders. Now it is necessary in my heart to love and care for these elders. They became *my* elders, *my family.* There was no doubt that this was a vocation, not an obligation. This is beautiful labor. It is spiritual. God helps me every day."

Another shared how getting to know the elders makes her happy: "I like to take care of elders. At first it was difficult; they were different, and I did not have experience. But I realized the elders were loving and affectionate. I have grown to cherish them. They make my day with what they talk about. They are brave. They are funny. I have fallen in love with them."

Caregivers talk about learning from elders, about the kindness, humor, and strength they see each day in their faces. Elders motivate the caregivers to learn more about themselves, to find patience, to develop skills they did not think they had, to be more conscientious, to be more centered. Elders inspire caregivers toward career paths in nursing, social work, medicine, and administration. Elders push caregivers to grow. Lao Tzu wrote, "Being deeply loved by someone gives you strength, while loving someone deeply gives you courage."

"I do this work because in the future I want to be a nurse," says a Vista caregiver. "I want to know how to care for people from the very beginning: cleaning them, showers, helping them eat, just being with elders. I want to be conscientious. This job is teaching me responsibility. If I want to have a medical career, I need to know what it is really like to care for someone who is really in need of care. I need to know what it means to help elders."

Honor, loss, and faith

Care and love are the connections between generations. All of our stories are expressed in either our ability or inability to care for others.

Heartbreak and loss change all of us. Many of us come into helping professions after living through pain. In the beginning of this book, there is the story of an elder who, in facing her own pain, makes the choice to help another elder. Caregivers follow this path as well. They often care for elders "in honor" of someone they loved and lost. This can be a parent, grandparent, child, partner, or friend. One of our caregivers spoke with tears in her eyes about how much reverence she has for eldercare and end-of-life care. She does this work in honor of her mother. She was far away from her mother when she died, unable to be with her. She expresses her grief through committing herself to caregiving; her healing comes from being present for others.

Another caregiver spoke of becoming a grandmother for the first time and how this reflected in her work: "I want to teach my children how to have patience. I want my grandchildren to love the elderly. I want them to share love with all their hearts."

One caregiver wrote of the deep connection her work has to her faith: "I like to help elders. Everything I do, I do with love. No regret. Someday I, or my family, or my children will need this help. I am getting older. I know that everything we do in this world because we are flesh and bones will return to dust. We are nothing until we rest our soul in life. God is love."

The thing that has always stayed with me from being a kid in church is this: God is love. You know how close you are to this love by how you treat the sick, the poor, and the suffering. Caregivers express this love each day in countless ways. "Dios es amor."

Remembering

Writing this, I find myself remembering, sorting through bits and pieces of all the beautiful words I have heard and the kindness I have seen. The work I have done is a gift, but like all true gifts, it is not easy. This work is love, and it is loss. Our job is to fall in love, stand by someone, and let them go. And then do it all over again.

I started working at Vista (before it was Vista) only a couple of months after Morgan moved in with me and after we lost our father. In recording the words of our caregivers, I remember my father; I hear his voice. His contradictions, his struggles, his faith, his sadness, and his love echo in the work I do. But while I live with the memory of my father, the ghost I have met in my work is my mother.

It was a cold, cloudy afternoon. I was helping a hospice nurse check on an elderly lady. She was beautiful, with big dark eyes, salt and pepper black hair, and a great smile. By then she was thin, tiny. She loved music, had raised an amazing family, and was tough and smart. As I helped her shift in her bed, she put one arm over my shoulder and, with her other hand, touched my face and smiled. In her dark eyes, something from decades earlier came back. The movement was a physical memory. I took a breath, helped the nurse, and held the elder's hand until she slept. I found myself in tears as I closed up for the day. I found myself sobbing that night as the memory came back. I realized I had been there before.

My mother died of cancer when I was eleven. She had fought it for four years. Cancer had aged her. At the end, she was thin, tiny. Her black hair had become salt and pepper. Her dark eyes seemed to be her whole face. On a cold winter evening, I helped lift her so she could read *The Phantom Tollbooth* to Morgan. I remember she struggled as she read. She put an arm over my shoulder, and it was easy to move her. She smiled, touched my cheek, and took the book. She would die a few days later, in the morning after Morgan and I were on the bus to school.

The elder we were caring for left our world. At her Rosary, there was a picture of her as she graduated high school. Before going to the service, I looked at our family Bible. My father had pasted a picture of Mom in the front cover, her college graduation picture. These two women who never knew each other and lived hundreds of miles apart were, in many ways, a distant mirror of each other. Until I was helping the elder move that day, I had not let myself see this. But listening to her family tell stories of her life, I realized these two women would have had many things in common—music, gardening, camping, toughness, stubbornness, and a deep love for family.

Many people who work with elders or in hospice care have similar stories. There is an understanding in counseling, social work, and art-therapy education programs that helpers end up working with the people who have the most to teach them. This often seems to be true. Palliative care was not what I wanted to do when I was in college, but this is where I have found my home. Caregivers in this work often come from cultures that respect the nurturing of others as an honored career choice, or from backgrounds that include elders in everyday life; they often have deep family histories of giving care. This influences their decisions to stay with the work. In my experience and in the stories I have heard from other caregivers, we meet ourselves in the people we help.

24/7

In 2015, AARP estimated that 39.8 percent of professional caregivers also care for a family member at home. In our own Vista ecosystem, the fact that the value of connection and care is in the DNA of so many of our staff has changed our way of working. The idea of care first/love rules is a natural expression of this. We share an innate belief that care, protection, and loving connection are the most important aspects of our work. Our nurse, Kris, described her DNA this way: "Strong urges to nurture all living things since childhood, unable to tolerate suffering, need to step in and try to help. It is time for light workers."

We try to make life better for elders *and* staff. We are as flexible as possible and make a conscious effort to accommodate staff needs around family care, even though it is complicated and imperfect. We are always a work in progress—our Vista Living Care system is dynamic. Vista is a living ecosystem, changing as needed to be healthy and adapting to changes in our greater communities. We try to be honest about whether we are providing the best possible care.

It is good to work in healthcare but not be owned by a healthcare company. It is good to have a structure that allows for changes and encourages new ideas. Much of the writing on burnout and compassion fatigue is focused on limitations. These limitations can include ideas, creativity, and even caring and connection, all of which can sever the link to being human. Systems that are set up to help human beings can become machines and forget the need to be human, thereby helping no one. An essential element of caregiving is paying attention. Machines can't pay attention to the often tiny but critical changes an elder may face on any given day. Systems that become fixed and mechanical can't see the often tiny but critical changes that happen with staff. Human beings who work as caregivers and then go home to be caregivers deserve an environment that cares for them. No one can be on 24/7. Human beings get tired. We need breathing room. Caregivers need systems that remember to be human, systems that are alive.

Maybe you can save the world, one person at a time

No caregiver, family, or professional can save someone from progressive dementia, and no home will be able to help every family that comes through their door. That said, we all have the responsibility to try to make life better whenever possible. We are called to tend, mend, fix, repair, and comfort. The call of caregiving is to value those who are forgotten, to push back on the pain of disease, to offer comfort when possible, and to stand by those who can't be comforted.

Our environmental director, Gary, described the work he does in this way: "I enjoy fixing and taking care of things that are broken, things—and people—that I can fix with my hands, my hands, my mind, or my heart." These words come from a man who is retired from a law-enforcement calling that spanned decades. Gary has seen plenty of "broken."

In Shelley E. Taylor's book *The Tending Instinct: How Nurturing Is Essential to Who We Are and How We Live*, she explores the biochemical, neurological, and evolutionary roots of nurturing. She concludes that caring for others is a deep need, an essential part of what makes us human. Tending, mending, fixing, and loving—the effort it takes to create and maintain a home and family—are all faces of that innate human need to care for others. I think as a society we forget how important it is to tend, mend, fix, and nurture. In more rigid institutional settings, this gets lost. But it is this deeper connection that makes life better for elders. Our Vista Living Care community works very hard to honor this connection.

This connection has to be part of the lives of everyone involved in care. Everyone. When it is lost, care suffers. When directors, CEOs, or administrators become separated from the hands-on work of providing care and creating a home, the situation becomes toxic for both the elders and the caregivers. Velma, our regional director, shared an experience of working in a setting where this connection to care was either completely severed or never existed to begin with:

"Many years ago, I took a part-time job out of college at a nursing home. I was assigned to the 'Alzheimer's unit' at the far back of the building, despite not knowing anything about Alzheimer's. The paint was peeling, the stench was appalling, and the elders' heads bent forward with nobody to talk to them. The long hallway with an unpolished floor led to a tiny, cluttered, L-shaped nurse's station, where the staff and the nurse chuckled at the elders. In a small multipurpose room to the right, with broken blinds and padlocks on the refrigerators, sat more elders, their clothing soiled from a previous meal, their hands dirty. One was searching for his cattle in the trashcan. I can close my eyes and still vividly see every wrinkle and whisker on his beautiful brown skin—his name was Margarito. Some elders in that room, not cognizant enough to lift a spoon, had plates in front of them filled with questionable portions of cold, chalky food. I will never forget this.

"To my own surprise I stuck it out, and my heart bled for them every day. As I became more and more intrigued by this disease, I requested to stay there. My grandfather had lived to a hundred years old, sharp as a tack, and the longevity of life on both sides of my family is healthy up into the late nineties. I was raised closely around the elderly in my family and in my small community of Questa, New Mexico. I told myself back then that if I were ever able to make a difference in the life of an institutionalized elder, I would. Sadly, my bucket of paint, the clothes from my mother's closet for the ladies, and curtains from the Goodwill weren't enough to make a difference in that setting. I became an avid advocate for the dignity and rights of the elders there, which was not well received by the corporate offices.

"As my grandfather would say, 'One door closes, another opens.' Twenty-one years ago, I applied for work at Vista Living Care and was hired on the spot. That was the turning point in my life, to be blessed with an owner who gave me the liberty to take care of the elders in an ethical, humane way. All these years later, over two decades, I am content and blessed to have more than fulfilled my commitment to the elders assigned to my care. There have been many ups, many downs, and blood, sweat, and tears. However, none of it would have been possible without the shared vision of owners Joe, Deb, and Luke Nachtrab and their family. I owe it all to them."

Directors, at least the really good ones, are caregivers. Caregivers want to care. Caregivers want to make life better for others. Caregivers want to protect families. Caregivers want to create warm, lovely homes. Caregivers need systems that encourage the desire to create a home. Caregivers do amazing work every day, even in situations that do not support their humanity, passion, or empathy. Caregivers fight bad systems; they bring in their own curtains and paint, they stay late or come in early to make life just a little bit better for the people they care for.

Sometimes, something wonderful happens. Now and then there is a situation where the values of caregivers and the values of owners, administrators, and systems match. Our Vista ecosystem is based on the values of family, love, and the unwavering commitment to make life better. This comes from the Nachtrab family. They have provided the support and space for all of us to grow. They have patiently stood by us caregivers through explorations ranging from murals to animals to the Eden Alternative and now to this book. All of these explorations have helped us grow and helped us create homes that are warm and alive. We have the space to be the caregivers we want to be because everyone is connected to care.

Velma came into this work as an advocate, a fierce fighter. She is still both. The blessing is that now she has people to join her. She gets to win. She gets to make a difference.

Healing

I came to this work differently. I came to this work hesitant and broken.

I finished graduate school in November of 1998 and was beginning the process of looking for work. During all the chaos of sending out resumes, making calls, applying for grants, running a cleaning business, and teaching classes, I realized I had not heard from my father. (Dad refused to have a phone after spending most of his adult life on call. He wrote letters.)

I called the sheriff in Cottage Grove, Oregon, where he and Morgan were living. I got a call back from the sheriff's office a few hours later on a cold, nasty evening. They had found Dad dead on the floor, with a blanket over him and a cold cup of tea next to him. He was building a bookcase when his heart stopped. Morgan, then thirty-one, was in his bedroom sitting on the bed, wrapped in blankets with his toys nearby. He was severely hypothermic and dehydrated, unable to speak or walk. Morgan was sent to a hospital in Eugene. The sheriff said the weather had been warm but turned cold about four days earlier. The windows were open in the house, and the heat was off. The coroner estimated that Dad had died more than a week before.

My (then) husband, Pepe, and I got a flight to Portland that left at 3 a.m. We drove to Eugene, where Pepe got us a room. I stayed with Morgan in the hospital. He was discharged the following day with orders to get physical therapy and see a cardiologist when we got back to Santa Fe. I made Dad's arrangements over the phone from the hotel while helping Morgan come back to the world. I fed him, showered him, pushed him to drink, and got him to take a few steps at a time. Cynthia, an old friend from Gallup, flew up two days later. She helped Pepe clean the house, replace the carpet, and find someone to sell the house. We found a walker and a wheelchair at a local thrift store.

After the house was cleaned, we took a day and drove to the beach. We walked on the beach with Morgan holding onto the two of us the whole time. He and Pepe found a squid tentacle and some whale bones. Morgan thought that was cool; he laughed and made a face. That was good to see. We rented a small U-Haul and drove back to Santa Fe with Morgan's furniture and toys.

Before we left, we put food and a salt block out for the deer that Dad had been in the habit of feeding. Cynthia burned sage. We tried to reach around a redwood out in the yard; holding hands, four adults could not reach around it. (I can hear Luke laughing about me hugging a tree as I write this.) I understood why Dad loved the place, but life for us was in Santa Fe. As we were leaving, I looked back and saw a deer in the driveway just watching us drive away.

This was the week of Thanksgiving. I stopped everything in my life other than getting Morgan settled, bringing him to doctor's appointments, setting up day programs, and starting physical therapy. Getting Morgan healthy and secure, and keeping him with us, was all that mattered. I got sick three times and paid for doctor visits by taking on housecleaning jobs and asking for antibiotic samples. Mostly, I just pushed through. The savings we had kept us above water for a little while. We managed to have a beautiful Christmas.

After the holidays, we started a routine for Morgan of day habilitation, therapy, and exercise to get him walking again. He reconnected with our cat, whom he had earlier named Angel Baby, which soon became just Baby. She sat with Morgan every afternoon while he watched *Star Wars*. They just hung out. Slowly, he started sleeping better, no longer waking up with nightmares. He also had more energy during the day. He cried, which was better than being shut down. Morgan enjoyed going to day hab three days a week. We were able to bring him back to a cozy, secure life. He very slowly became more independent.

I went back to teaching art classes at Open Hands, a local adult day program. The director there introduced me to Casa Pacifica, which would eventually evolve into Sierra Vista, the first of the Vista Living Care homes. She said, "It is a little place down the street. They could use your energy. I know you're looking for full time, but I think you could really help the seniors there while you are looking."

Casa Pacifica was owned by an RN who had for years tried to run a home for fifteen elders with minimal staff, money, and energy. The home and everyone in it was drifting.

Though I was working with dementia at Open Hands, I knew little about frailty. I had never worked in a nursing home and had only visited one once in my life. Our church took cookies and sang carols at a nursing home one Christmas when I was in middle school. I remembered the smell—Casa Pacifica smelled like that. I had also worked in the mental health field, with addicts and inmates. I had been around restrictive, cold, and at times scary environments, but never in a sad one. This was a sad place at the time.

I got hired to teach art classes and was turned loose to "cheer up the seniors" for ten hours a week. I brought in paint, collage paper, books, old movies, music, and new couch covers. For two hours, five days a week, I got to know the elders there. After you woke them up and started talking to them, they were amazing. Nita loved color and laughed a lot, though she could not talk. David was cynical, ornery, and cursed like a sailor, but he was also really wonderful. Dorothy and Millie were inseparable and were both great dancers. Verna loved red nail polish though her husband hated it. My ten hours ended up being twenty or more, often unpaid. But there was flexibility, which I needed in order to care for Morgan and deal with selling Dad's house.

About a month after I began working at Casa Pacifica, I noticed a rather large bump under my left collarbone. I figured I had just pulled a muscle. I iced it, but it was a little sore. I tried to ignore it, but Pepe and my friend Linda were worried. They bugged me to see the doctor, finally making me an appointment at a women's health clinic. A friend, another Linda, went with me to make sure I went. I did not have insurance and really didn't have the money to mess with what I thought was nothing.

The doctor at the clinic did a breast exam and asked questions about my general health and history. When she heard my family history around cancer, and that I had had two sinus infections and the flu in the previous two months, she had my blood drawn and made me wait in the office for "stat" results. This took almost three hours, which was annoying. When the bloodwork came in, the doctor looked at the results, frowned, and shook her head. She made an appointment for a diagnostic mammogram the following day.

I ended up in another doctor's office the following afternoon with that doctor calling a surgeon for a biopsy. Stat. That was Friday. I saw the surgeon on Monday. On Wednesday afternoon, a biopsy was done on the bump and on the lymph nodes under my left arm.

I got a call the following Monday while Morgan was getting ready for day hab and I was printing resumes. It was cancer, large mass, very aggressive, with probable lymph involvement. I needed to be in surgery at 6 a.m. on Thursday. I punched a wall, helped Morgan pack his lunch, and took him to day hab. I made arrangements to miss work in both places for two to three weeks and cancelled my housecleaning jobs for the month. That evening, I sat down with Pepe and Linda, figured out Morgan's schedule, and finally cried.

That day, just eight days after my initial doctor's appointment, would start the blur that brings cancer into this story. Honestly, I was more angry than afraid. Cancer felt like a roadblock in the way of my getting on with life. Initially, cancer just irritated me. Caring for Morgan had basically made Pepe and me parents overnight. He was just beginning to get settled, and Pepe and I were trying to be okay. I started the process of applying for waiver programs to help pay for Morgan's day programs as our savings were dropping fast. (It would end up taking more than a decade to find a situation that really worked for Morgan's medical and financial life, but that is another story.)

The surgery went well. The recovery took a couple of weeks, with a drain under my arm and orders for physical therapy that I ended up blowing off because I didn't have insurance. I left the hospital the day after surgery with no lymph nodes on my left side, a five-inch cut above my left breast and muscle, and with tissue and tendons removed from my chest. I would also leave the hospital with more than $10,000 in debt. That was just the beginning.

Three weeks later we sat down with the oncologist, Dr. Tim Lopez, to discuss the follow-up. I remember thinking it was strange—we were all about the same age, in our early thirties, too young to be talking cancer.

Follow-up meant high-dose chemotherapy, radiation, and ta-moxifen. I resisted. "Can't it wait until I'm working full-time? I don't have insurance. We don't have any money left. What would happen if I just waited a couple of months, maybe three?"

The answer was simple, given first in English for me and then in Spanish for Pepe: "You could die." The doctor said, "Some things just suck, but we will beat this. You have to deal with this now. If you wait till you can afford this, you will die." That conversation ended up saving my life. It also ended up being my model for how to talk to families from that point on. Yes, this sucks, but we will be there. This sucks, but that's okay.

I started chemo the following Friday. It was okay. I took med-icine for the nausea. I slept all weekend and woke up Monday pretty foggy and weak, but the next day I was back teaching my art groups. I remember thinking, I got this—no problem. However, I did, at Pepe and Linda's request, back off on the job search. That ended up being wise advice.

Life was pretty normal. I was frustrated with Casa Pacifica and was doing tasks like cleaning, changing Depends, and brushing teeth. All of that would have earned me a good Dr. Lopez lecture, but oh well. Casa Pacifica did hire two care-givers, Lety and Rosenda, who were interested in the elders and their care. I think all three of us realized we simply could only get so far, but we tried.

My next round of chemo was the week before Mother's Day. When I got back to Casa Pacifica, we started doing our best to clean and pretty up for a party. Rosenda worked really hard on the living room carpet with a mop and scrubber. We made paper flowers, brought in bright colored serapes for the couches, and put up streamers. It may not have been elegant, but at least it was colorful. When I was walking down the hall with one of the elders, I heard a shriek in Spanish that I'm pretty glad I couldn't understand. There was a trail of hair on the newly cleaned carpet. My hair. We cleaned it up and I went home and shaved my head.

We had the party the following day. An elder's daughter brought two dozen roses. I got some money from the facility for a little champagne, sparkling cider, strawberries, and chocolates. One of the caregivers brought a fruit salad. We celebrated. One of the ladies kept taking off my hat and rubbing my head. Another got three different staff members to pour her champagne. It was a good day, and I was tired.

Tired became a normal part of life, as did many strange little things: The smell of Colgate toothpaste made me want to throw up, bright lights gave me headaches, I got motion sickness, noise bothered me, and my body felt like a weird stranger. To do a round of chemo, you have to get blood drawn to make sure your immune system is functioning. The first two rounds were pretty ordinary, but June was different. My chemo ended up being pushed back three weeks.

Next we did Father's Day at Casa Pacifica. A gentleman's son, daughter-in-law, and I pulled weeds in the back and set up a badminton net. I kept sneaking to the bathroom to throw up and brush my teeth, but we ended up with a workable yard for a barbeque. The son brought his grill, a caregiver brought beans, and Pepe dropped off burgers, green chile, and cheese from the restaurant he managed. The food looked good. The elders ate well. We played no-rules badminton. The following week, I was able to do chemo again.

That round of chemo was just bad. A vein collapsed while the chemo drugs were being delivered. This left me with a nasty red scar that looked a lot like track marks running from my right palm to my elbow. The usual routine of sleeping for a couple of days, feeling rotten for a day, and then going back to life ended up taking more than a week. I developed some kind of secondary infection, spiked a fever, and got a shot of antibiotics and more pills. There was a lot of vomiting and general unpleasantness. There was also fatigue that just stayed around after everything else was finished. Cancer had become the dominant force in my life.

By the time I got back to work, the building had been sold to Sierra Vista, and Casa Pacifica was no more. I was basically okay with that. There had been rumors for months about the owner retiring and selling.

I also learned that two elders had died, which was hard. Awful, actually.

I had called in while I was out sick but did not get through to anyone and just did not have the energy to keep trying. It turned out the owner of Casa Pacifica had not passed the staffing list along, so when I showed up, I was a surprise. And not a good one. I met Velma, our new director, on July 1. She looked a bit shell shocked—well-dressed, but shell shocked. Velma told me later that in addition to all the work the building would need, she thought I looked like a heroin addict. I was thin (not a natural state for me) and bald, with a scar running up my right arm and dark circles around my eyes. I used colorful cloth hats to cover my head because wigs made me miserable. Pepe and Linda kept telling me I looked great, but they were just being cheerleaders.

The July Fourth holiday gave me a purpose. I tossed out the idea of a banana split party, figuring that a barbeque might make me sick. Ed, our regional director at the time, and Velma went for the idea because of its simplicity.

As Ed and I took a drive to Albertson's for ice cream, toppings, and party favors, we ended up having a discussion that would change the course of my life. I told him the truth: I was sick. Cancer, late stage three. I lifted my sleeve and took off my hat. I had every intention of looking for another job when I finished treatment. The facility was a mess; we both agreed on that. Ed wanted to turn activities into a full-time job to make life better for the elders. I figured it was only a matter of time before I was out of a job. I also figured I didn't have anything to lose, so I just put out an idea: I was willing to go full-time after treatment if I could get health insurance. Money didn't matter.

There was no way for me to work full-time until after treatment. There were more rounds of chemo scheduled, plus radiation. I had an appointment the following week to have a port put into my chest that would allow me to keep taking chemo after the vein broke. There was a pretty good chance that that broken vein would turn into another infection and require surgery. The bills were just coming in and going into a pile. I had applied for the indigent fund at the hospital, but that only covered part of the expenses, and that was already spent. In total, the treatment for my cancer would take fourteen months.

My work at Open Hands was funded through a Community Arts grant, and leaving was not an option. The grant money followed the artist. I was, for better or worse, that artist. Morgan was steady, but he had started to become tired, at times short of breath and with occasional swelling in his feet. We had an appointment for him to see a cardiologist. I felt like a storm was out there somewhere, waiting for Morgan. Thinking back, everything and everyone connected to the new Sierra Vista building at that time was complicated.

There is a term in cancer care called "nadir." The nadir is the point when someone's body and immune system are at their lowest, the most frail. Nadir is the point of greatest danger. It is the point when the most cancer cells are being cleared, the point when new life and health can begin. Nadir is also the point when one can lose the fight and die. I was in nadir. But I was not alone. The building, the elders, the caregivers and their families were also in nadir.

Limping through like Casa Pacifica had been doing for a long time was no longer an option; it was just too toxic. We were all in a place with only two choices: Heal and live, or lose and die. My nadir was physical. The elders, families, staff, and building faced a nadir in spirit, learning how to live instead of just existing. To live for all of us would mean fighting, taking shaky, slow, often painful steps back to being alive.

Ed, Velma, and the Nachtrab family faced choices that hot July. They could clear out the staff and start over, or they could commit to the slow, stressful path of trying to mend what was there. They chose the latter. Why, I am not sure, but they did. They also took me up on the full-time-after-treatment-for-insurance idea. I am not sure why. This choice would change the course of not only my life for a very long time, but also the lives of the elders, the families, and the two caregivers who came in at the same time I did. That choice would help me live. There would still be a long fight, but there was also a turn toward embracing life. That choice would begin a transformation for the home and everyone in it. It would be a slow, hard process of healing, growing, and remodeling. It would also be fun.

First there would be paint, carpet, beds, and furniture. During this process, I would learn that the neglect at Casa Pacifica was deeper than I had allowed myself to see. There were mice; bad plumbing, heating and cooling issues, and many other problems small and large. Becoming functional took time. But it was a wonderful experience, from my point of view. Life was coming back into the home. Each day there was a little more strength, a few more smiles, a little more hope. I learned something then: Transformation is not a lightning bolt, a sudden dramatic event; it is slower, more sensible. It is day to day. A coat of paint, homemade bread and chicken soup in the kitchen, fresh-smelling sheets, the feeling of being a little less tired at the end of a day, learning all the words to "Frankie and Johnny," ordering art supplies, a survey with perfect results, a daughter-in-law telling you how she and her husband felt safe enough to go away for their thirtieth anniversary because Dad was okay—all these things were transformative.

Of course there were also struggles and loss: four divorces, including my own; caring for an elder whom we were unable to comfort despite all love and effort; beloved staff leaving to follow new paths; struggles with balancing professional and family caregiving; and the bittersweet, intense connection that comes from standing with elders through dementia. Velma and I have both had to adapt. We have had to learn about trust and humility as our roles have changed.

Laughter, friendship, growth, tough choices, great ideas, experiments that did or didn't work, and some beautiful, fierce miracles all become the soil for our odd, little ecosystem. Velma got married in 2018, and Morgan served as a groomsman. There were times when this event seemed completely impossible. Velma lives the miracle of being able to open her heart and life to a man who loves her, and her husband, Kevin, is open to her beautiful, noisy, complicated family. Her miracle has been a slow, quiet, day-to-day, very human miracle.

Morgan's life is a miracle. The fact that he is strong enough to walk down a church aisle is a miracle. For the past year and a half, he has been able to live his life on his schedule. He rests when he needs to. It's okay that it takes two to three hours to get ready for the day. He enjoys music, movies, Flor the cat, Honey the dog, and new cafes. His life is based on joy and simplicity. We keep what gives him joy and comfort and let go of the rest. He is prayed for; he is loved. He gives love; he prays for others. He is independent in some ways and needs help in others. Everything is part of life. Someday his heart will stop. That is part of life too. But right now I am blessed with the miracle that is Morgan.

The joy, simplicity, and clarity of Morgan's life and the complicated, tangled decisions that went into creating that life also show in our shared vision for his other family that is Vista Living Care. The connection to others, the respect for a life that is simple and joyful, is what we all want for our elders. The elders we work with are like Morgan, past much of the nonsense that we "normal" people get lost in. They live in a place that is much deeper, much more real, and in many ways more clear than the rest of the world. We get to share this. Our job is to create and maintain a place for these amazing human beings to simply be who they are. Our job is to create the place where joy and comfort can live. Our place is also to let go of the rest.

Care first, love rules

It is funny that when we look at elder homes, we don't spend much time talking about what really makes a home. We talk about fixtures, amenities, staffing, emergency protocols, technology, and equipment. This conversation needs to change. A home is made or destroyed by the people in it. I am not opposed to great fixtures or to technology—they can be great tools in the right hands. But these things, no matter how fascinating they may be, do not make a home. Things are not a relationship. They are not a connection to life. Homes evolve over time to reflect the people who live there. Homes change. Home is where people feel safe. Home is where you can be exactly who you are.

Maybe our conversations about eldercare should begin with relationships. Do caregivers feel heard when they have concerns? Do they know the elders not as diagnoses, room numbers, or occupancy, but as human beings? Is there a deep commitment to the day-to-day, hands-on care that someone facing dementia will need, or is that care a reason to increase fees? Is Alzheimer's being discussed in an honest way, or is the structure of the entire system built on catering to denial? The relationship between someone who needs help and someone who gives help is complex. This relationship can be human and loving and enrich both people's lives, or it can be mechanical and neglectful.

Carol, our executive director at Vista Living Care, describes her vision of care like this: "Love connects us all. We draw our strength from the energy we create together. I love doing this work because our differences make us look for similarities in one another. No matter how broken we may feel, there is strength in coming together that makes us whole again. Caregiving completes me."

The day-to-day relationships among elders, caregivers, families, friends, and the community are what is important to the Vista Living Care ecosystem. The only rule is love. The most important commitment is caring. Carol's description reminds me of the aspen forest in the beginning of this book. It is the connection, the tangled roots, that matters. To be strong in the face of any life-threatening challenge, we need each other. Pretty, perfect boxes don't care for people; people do. The aspens survive wind, cold, rain, drought, heat, and snow. They stand by one another growing from shared roots. Some die while others sprout and grow. Elders live with beauty in the face of pain and death. Caregivers stand, hold the space, and give care. Something beautiful happens, something real and beautiful.

Epilogue: An Unfinished Story

Two elderly ladies sit with a caregiver in a bright, cozy dining room looking at glossy coffee-table books of mountain scenery and roses, deciding where they want to travel. They snack on homemade sugar cookies and cider.

One gentleman goes off to church with his son and daughter-in-law, bringing home even more cookies. Another gentleman goes out to volunteer at the college radio station with his helper and friend, Yolanda, whom he describes as "more beautiful than Silver." (Silver is a German shepherd at one of our homes.) Our house smells like lavender and cinnamon, with a tiny bit of remodeling dust mixed in. Morgan is watching *A Christmas Carol* with Robert, celebrating their love of movies and soda. A caregiver is helping Norma fold clothes. Loyce opens presents and drinks eggnog with her daughter and granddaughter. Maybe later we all will look at paint samples for the walls or trim the last bowl from pottery class or do a bit of stretching to balance out some of the cookies and chocolate.

One of the places where the ladies looking at books want to go is the aspen forest outside of Taos, in Northern New Mexico. Older, taller trees stand near smaller saplings, all of them clad in leaves of the brightest yellow-gold. This home, Vista Hermosa, is a sapling in our Vista ecosystem. There are people here who face dementia and people who remember everything but need other supports. We are focused enough and intimate enough to do both. Elders can give support to others as well as receive support.

On the way here, I caught the last few sentences of a news story about deaths at a nursing home following a hurricane in Florida. The talk was about penalties, but nothing about how to really change the system that allowed this tragedy to happen. After hearing this I walked into Vista Hermosa, a bright house with plants, pets, and people who are connected to one another, nurtured, and loved. Our Vista ecosystem gives me hope. There is potential here, creativity and life.

Josef Beuys, a German artist, gave different responses when asked what work of art he was most proud of: One was his engagement in social change, another was teaching, and the last, as he was dying of cancer, was his marriage. These answers were a way of expressing that all life well lived is a creative process with infinite potential. Life itself is art.

In Velma's words, our hope is to "have a completely different conversation" about aging and care. This conversation is about growth, life, and hope. This conversation is about care and love.

About the Authors

Ruth Dennis

R uth has worked in mental health, the arts, and community education for more than twenty-five years. She is a Certified Dementia Practitioner and for the past two decades has worked closely with and researched palliative care, hospice, and grief support. She has counseled and taught in recovery programs and in transitional homes that serve homeless mentally ill adults, developmentally disabled adults, and elders facing dementia.

Ruth earned a master's degree in art therapy from Southwestern College in Santa Fe, N.M.; she earned a master of fine arts degree in ceramics from Cranbrook Academy of Art; and she earned a master of fine arts degree, independent study in architecture, also from Cranbrook Academy of Art. She has been an artist in residence with the Bemis Foundation, South Carolina Arts in the Schools, and Rehoboth McKinley Christian Hospital. She has also worked with grants funded by the National Endowment for the Arts and others.

Ruth has presented at the International Eden Alternative Conference, the National Art Therapy Association Conference, the New Mexico State Agency on Aging, the New Mexico Chapter of the Alzheimer's Association, and many other statewide educational conferences.

Central to Ruth's life is her role as caregiver to her brother Morgan, who has Down Syndrome. He is the bravest man she has ever known.

Velma Arellano

Velma Arellano has been working in elder care for more than two decades. She has overseen $2 million in construction to create, design, remodel, and scheme two state-of-the-art Alzheimer's memory care homes in New Mexico. Both homes are currently the only two Eden Alternative Registered homes in New Mexico.

Velma is a Certified Assisted Living Administrator and a Certified Dementia Practitioner through the National Council of Certified Dementia Practitioners. She has received recognition in New Mexico for her commitment to improving the lives of elders by placing love, care, and fun before business models, and to truly changing the culture of how we care for our aging institutionalized population. Velma has served on the board of the New Mexico Alzheimer's Association and was instrumental in the passage of Helen's Law, which protects endangered elders.

Velma's current venture is Vista Hermosa, an intimate assisted living home specializing in the care of elders who need minimal to moderate assistance with daily living. Vista Hermosa is drawing on the cutting edge of the culture of change by researching and incorporating the ideas of permaculture, sustainability, organics, natural medicine, aromatherapy, and many other movements for positive change in long-term elder care.

A proud native of Northern New Mexico, Velma has served on the board of the 305th annual *Concilio de la Fiesta de Santa Fe* and belongs to century-old Roman Catholic societies. As an active rancher, she is a member of the Llano Irrigation Ditch Company, which was established in the mid-1800s. Velma is a member of ECO, the Earth Citizens Organization. She also practices brain yoga, a Korean modality founded by the renowned Ilchi Lee.

Velma earned a master's degree in agency counseling and psychology from New Mexico Highlands University, and a bachelor's degree in television broadcast journalism/mass communication and Spanish, also from New Mexico Highlands University.

Velma is honored to have cared for her lovely 85-year old mother, Mary, in the last year of her life until she succumbed from cancer, after having fought and beat it several times in her life.

Luke Nachtrab

Luke Nachtrab is an owner and the president of Vista Living. He and his wife, Kara, have three children—Joey, Kate, and Molly—and live in Sylvania, Ohio, where the Vista Living Home Office is based.

Shortly after earning his undergraduate degree at The Ohio State University, Luke became the first employee of Northaven, the Nachtrab family's business management company. In 2004, when Northaven assumed operations of Vista Living from his father, Luke's passion and love for the elderly, particularly those walking with forgetfulness, began to flourish. He was named president of Vista Living Communities in 2011, and in 2014 set the company up for growth. His passion for making a positive impact on those with dementia and their families is evident in his business philosophy, where integrity and compassion come first.

Luke has a diverse business background, but his passion lies with Vista Living. He has served on numerous boards in the Toledo area, including his current post at St. John's Jesuit High School. He is also active in Argentum and their mission to expand senior living.

In an effort toward continuous improvement, Luke has completed many non-degree courses, and in 2011 earned his MBA from the University of Michigan Ross School of Business. He is an instrument-rated pilot and loves skiing, golfing, soccer, squash, fishing, culture, traveling, watching the Buckeyes, and being a dad! He looks forward to raising his children to some-day be involved with the business.

Resources and References

Helpful Reading

Anything by these authors:
Larry Dossey, M.D.
Atul Gawande, M.D.
Gary Glazner, M.A.
G. Allen Power, M.D.
Teepa Snow, M.S.
Richard Taylor, PhD.
William Thomas, M.D.

Books

Alcoholics Anonymous: 75th Anniversary Edition Blue Book

Cope, Denys. *Dying: A Natural Passage.* Three Whales Publishing, 2008.

Coste, Joanne Koenig and Robert Buller. *Learning to Speak Alzheimer's: A Groundbreaking Approach for Everyone Dealing with the Disease.* Mariner Books, 2004.

Dossey, Larry. *The Extra-ordinary Healing Power of Ordinary Things: Fourteen Natural Steps to Health and Happiness.* Harmony, 2007.

Healey, Francie. *Eat to Beat Alzheimer's.* Terra Nova Books, 2016.

Hudson, Robert B., ed. *The New Politics of Old Age Policy, 3rd Edition.* Johns Hopkins University Press, 2014.

Huffington, Arianna. *The Sleep Revolution: Transforming Your Life, One Night at a Time.* Harmony, 2017.

Levine, Robert. *Defying Dementia: Understanding and Preventing Alzheimer's and Related Disorders.* Rowman and Littlefield Publishers, 2010.

Lokvig, Jytte Fogh. *The Alzheimer's Creativity Project: The Caregiver's Ultimate Guide to a Good Day; Communication and Activities in the World of Alzheimer's.* Self-published, 2014.

Maslach, Christina, and Philip G. Zimbardo. *Burnout: The Cost of Caring.* Malor Books, 2003.

Mc Namara, Norman, and Mrs. Elaine Waddington. *The Lewy Body Soldier.* CreateSpace Independent Publishing Platform, 2016.

National Geographic. "Your Brain: A User's Guide." National Geographic, 2018.

Power, Allen G. *Dementia Beyond Drugs.* Health Professions Press, 2010.

——— *Dementia Beyond Disease: Enhancing Well-Being.* Health Professions Press, 2016.

Ramachandran, V.S. *The Tell-Tale Brain: A Neuroscientist's Quest for What Makes Us Human.* W.W. Norton & Company, 2012.

Roszak, Theodore. *The Making of an Elder Culture: Reflections on the Future of America's Most Audacious Generation.* New Society Publishers, 2009.

Snyder, Pat. *Treasures in the Darkness Extending the Early Stage of Lewy Body Dementia, Alzheimer's, and Parkinson's Disease.* CreateSpace Independent Publishing Platform, 2012.

Taylor, Shelley E. *The Tending Instinct: How Nurturing Is Essential to Who We Are and How We Live.* Times Books, 2002.

Thomas, William. *What Are Old People For? How Elders Will Save the World.* Vanderwyk & Burnham, 2004.

Westheimer, Ruth, and Pierre A. Lehu. *Dr. Ruth's Guide for the Alzheimer's Caregiver How to Care for Your Loved One Without Getting Overwhelmed...and Without Doing It All Yourself.* Quill Driver Books, 2012.

Groups and Internet Resources

AARP
www.aarp.org
https://www.aarp.org/content/dam/aarp/ppi/2015/caregiving-in-the-united-states-2015-report-revised.pdf

Alzforum
www.alzforum.org/news/research-news/
brain-atrophy-patterns-support

Alzheimer's and Dementia Weekly
http://www.alzheimersweekly.com/2014/10/25-ways-to-mend-memory.html

Alzheimer's Association
https://www.alz.org

Alzheimer's Poetry Project
www.alzpoetry.com

Awakening from Alzheimer's
www.awakeningfromalzheimers.com

Centers for Disease Control
www.cdc.gov

Eden Alternative
www.edenalt.org

The Elder Consult Geriatric Medicine and Education website.
http://www.elderconsult.com/dementia-medications/

Global Deterioration Scale (Barry Reisberg, M.D.)
https://www.fhca.org/members/qi/clinadmin/global.pdf

Hogewyek Dementia Village
https://hogeweyk.dementiavillage.com/en/

Howard Kirschner, M.D.
https://emedicine.medscape.com/article/1135164-overview

Ibasho Elder Care
www.ibasho.org/web

MedicAlert + Alzheimer's Association's Safe Return
https://www.medicalert.org/safereturn

National Alzheimer's Project Act
https://aspe.hhs.gov/national-alzheimers-project-act

National Caregiving Alliance
www.caregiving.org

National Institute on Aging
www.nia.nih.gov

National Institutes of Health
www.nih.gov/
www.nia.nih.gov/health/
alzheimers-disease-people-down-syndrome
www.ncbi.nlm.nih.gov/pmc/articles/PMC4991646/
www.ncbi.nlm.nih.gov/pubmed/16889103

Dennis, Ruth. "Just another Love Story," *Natural Awakenings Magazine.* Natural Awakenings, Feb. 2013.

Patricia Gerbarg, M.D.
www.breath-body-mind.com/lyme-disease.php

Paying For Senior Care
https://www.payingforseniorcare.com/alzheimers/
financial-assistance.html

The Permaculture Movement
https://permacultureprinciples.com/flower/health

Prescribers' Digital Reference
www.pdr.net/

Public Broadcasting Services "Alzheimer's: Every Minute Counts" 25 Jan. 2017
https://www.pbs.org/show/alzheimers-every-minute-counts/

60 *Minutes* with Leslie Stahl, 27 Nov. 2016
https://www.cbsnews.com/news/
60-minutes-alzheimers-disease-medellin-colombia-lesley-stahl/

Teepa Snow, M.S.,
www.teepasnow.com

UC Irvine Memory Impairments and Neurological Disorders Research Institute
www.mind.uci.edu/

UC San Francisco
https://memory.ucsf.edu/art-creativity

http://www.neuroscience.ucsf.edu/neurograd/files/
ns245winter11/021611PERUSE_VBM_FTD_SD_common.pdf

UNM Memory and Aging Center
https://hsc.unm.edu/health/patient-care/neurosciences-
stroke-care/memory-aging-center.html

U.S. Bureau of Labor Statistics, 2018
https://www.bls.gov/ooh/healthcare/home-health-aides-and-
personal-care-aides.htm

U.S. Department of Labor
www.bls.gov/ooh/healthcare/home.htm

U.S. Department of Health and Human Services
www.ahcancal.org/quality_improvement/
Documents/UnderstandingDirectCareWorkers.pdf

World Health Organization
http://www.who.int/ageing/publications/global_health.pdf